I0757292

Intermittent Fasting and Ketogenic Diet

An Essential Guide to IF and Keto, Including Amazing Tips for Activating Autophagy and for Getting Into Ketosis

Contents

Part 1: Intermittent Fasting

How to Lose Weight, Burn Fat, and Increase Mental Clarity without Having to Give up All Your Favorite Foods

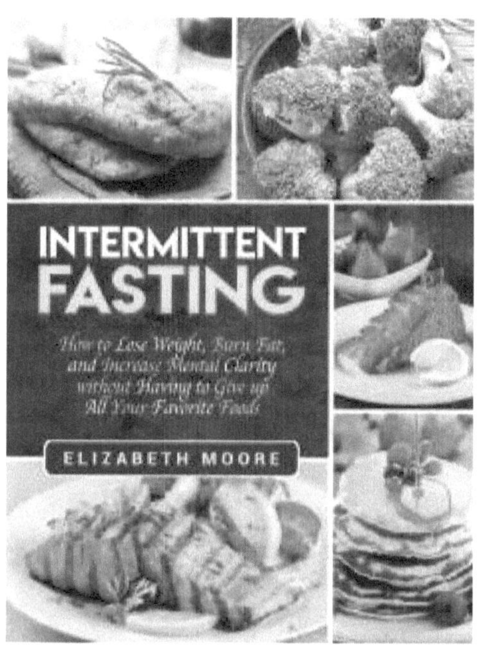

Introduction

With all the different types of dieting plans out there, it can sometimes be difficult to know which one is the best option. Some people like the idea of the ketogenic diet and eating good fats to promote lots of fat loss. Others like to go on a diet plan that helps them lower their blood pressure and reduce their salt intake. Then there are options that are low fat and higher carb, options for cleansing, and so much more. But which one is the best to choose?

This guidebook is going to spend some time looking at intermittent fasting and all the benefits that can come from following this eating plan. Intermittent fasting encourages healthy eating and puts a limit on the processed and junk foods that are common in the American diet. However, more importantly, intermittent fasting focuses on changing the way, and the times, that you eat.

The idea is to allow the body to go on short-term fasts during the week. This can help clean out the body, speed up the metabolism, and naturally help you to cut down on the number of calories that you consume during the week. And since there are different options when it comes to the type of intermittent fast you can go on, you are sure to find a method that works best for you.

This guidebook provides everything you need to know to get started with intermittent fasting. We will explore what intermittent fasting is, how to get started, some of the different methods that go with an intermittent fast, and some of the benefits and side effects that come with this kind of eating plan. Intermittent fasting may be a different way of eating, but it is going to provide you with some amazing benefits.

While the ideas behind fasting are pretty simple to follow, it is a great way to improve almost every aspect of your health. In addition to helping you lose weight and belly fat, an intermittent fast can help you burn fat, fight off some types of cancer, reduce your insulin levels, help keep the mind sharp, fight off and prevent diabetes, and so much more. All it takes is adjusting the times that you eat during the day.

Intermittent fasting has proven to be effective in helping so many people lose weight and feel better. While some of the results are similar to what can be done with continuous calorie restriction, intermittent fasting is often easier to follow than the latter and can even help you maintain more of your lean muscle mass in the process.

Take some time to read through this guidebook and learn everything that you need to know about intermittent fasting!

Chapter 1: What Is Intermittent Fasting?

While there are many different diet plans, one method that is often more effective at helping you work on your health and lose weight is intermittent fasting. This method can do so much for your body, and the ideas behind it are pretty simple.

With intermittent fasting, you need to concentrate on eating healthy and wholesome foods, but there aren't strict requirements on the foods that you eat. With this option, you will focus more on separating your day into two periods, one for eating and one for fasting or abstaining for eating. The second time period, your fasting window, needs to be longer than normal to help you better control your eating habits and the calories that you take in each day to improve your health.

Intermittent fasting and the different methods that go with it have grown in popularity. With all the great health benefits and the relative ease in which people lose weight on this eating plan, it is no wonder that everyone wants to give it a try. Let's take a look at some of the basics that you should know about intermittent fasting before moving on to discuss the benefits, how to get started, and so much more!

The History of Fasting

Fasting is not a new idea. It has been around for thousands of years. Pythagoras extolled the virtues of fasting, St. Catherine of Siena practiced fasting, and Paracelsus, a doctor during the Renaissance period, called fasting a "physician within" all of us. Fasting, in one form or another, is a distinguished tradition, and throughout the centuries, those who follow it claim that fasting can bring spiritual and physical renewal.

In primitive cultures, a fast would be needed before people went to war. It was also considered a coming of age ritual in many cultures. If the people were worried about an angry deity, a fast was often required, and North Americans would do it as a ceremony to avoid issues like famine.

Many of the major religions in the world have implemented fasting as part of their rituals. It can be used as a form of self-control and penitence or enacted for major events within the religion. For example, Judaism has several fasting days each year, including the Day of Atonement and Yom Kippur. In Islam, followers fast during the month of Ramadan. Easter orthodoxy and Roman Catholics will observe a 40-day fast during Lent.

While fasting has been commonly associated with religious and cultural practices in the past, there are times when fasting was used for other things as well. For example, it has often been used as a political protest tool. Mahatma Gandhi and the Suffragettes went under 17 fasts during the struggle for independence for India.

During the 19th century, a practice that is known as therapeutic fasting became popular to prevent illnesses and even treat some when they were done under medical supervision. This became something that grew with the Natural Hygiene Movement and is still popular today. This was seen as a natural way to help clean out the body and prevent illnesses without having to worry so much about taking medicines that could cause many side effects and harm the body.

Today, there are many reasons why someone would choose to go on a fast. They may choose to do it as a part of their religion, to protest something that they are against, or as a way to clean out their bodies and help them lose weight. Fasting has a long history and many different uses, which makes it the perfect choice when you are ready to make some changes in your diet and lifestyle.

The Basics of an Intermittent Fast

Intermittent fasting is less about the foods that you eat – although these can be important – and more about the timing of your meals. With a traditional American diet, you can easily eat nonstop during the day. Many people start with breakfast, have a snack around midmorning, lunch, another snack, a big dinner, and even another snack before bedtime. There are even some healthy eating plans that recommend eating five or six times a day to help you lose weight.

What all these end up doing is allowing us to eat way too many calories during the day. We are feeding the body a constant supply of energy in the form of glucose, but most of it is not being used and is then stored as extra body fat over time. We get into a bad cycle of eating a bunch of carbs and calories, but still wanting more. This cycle is going to cause us to gain weight and a whole host of other health conditions.

With intermittent fasting, you aim to change this cycle. You will learn how to limit your eating windows, not allowing yourself to eat all the time. This can help you reduce how much you take in and can naturally lead to weight loss. There are different options with intermittent fasting. Some ask you to go 24 hours without eating, some ask you to have a few days a week only eating 500 calories, and others ask you to do smaller fasts each day, limiting your eating window to eight hours or so.

No matter which method you choose to go with, you are limiting the amount of time that you can eat during the day. This results in fewer calories, easier weight loss, and more time to enjoy life. Think of all the freedom you will get just by cutting out a few of the meals that you have to plan and make each week!

When you go on an intermittent fast, you will need to consider what diet plan to go on. Many people like the ketogenic diet because it helps increase the fat burning that comes with fasting. However, many other diet plans can work with intermittent fasting as well. Don't try to start without a diet plan. There isn't one diet plan associated with fasting, but if you continue to take in too many calories and eat junk, you are going to have a hard time seeing results on your fast.

There are also different methods that you can choose when it comes to which type of intermittent fast you want. Some people like to go on an alternate day fast. Some like to have a few days a week, and they are really busy anyway when they fast. Others like to have shorter fasts added into each day. All these methods can be effective; you just need to choose the one that fits into your schedule and stick with it.

Do I Need to Worry About Starvation Mode?

One common concern about intermittent fasting is that you will quickly put your body into starvation mode if you try this form of eating. The worry is that these small fasts are going to be enough to ruin the metabolism and make it hard to lose weight or even function properly. The biggest issue here is that this concern is based on the idea that our bodies can't handle any stress, and going even a few hours without food can send it all out of order.

This is not true.

Think back to our ancestors. Did they have a constant stream of food at their disposal? Did they have horrible metabolic effects when they had to go a few days without eating because of famine or because the food was hard to come by? No, their bodies and ours were adapted to handle these shorter times without food to help them, and us, survive.

Starvation mode happens when you go a long time without food. The body starts to recognize that it isn't getting the nutrition that it once did, and so it will slow down the metabolism to keep you alive. However, studies show that it takes 72 hours or more before you start to see this occur. Intermittent fasting usually lasts less than 24 hours in a row. A few go up to 36 hours, but that is all.

These fasts are not going to be long enough even to come close to the body going into starvation mode. Instead, during these short fasts, the body is going to spend time speeding up the metabolism, burning more calories as it goes through your readily available glucose and then moving on to the glycogen stores as well. Since the fast is so short, and with you concentrating on eating wholesome and nutritious foods during your eating windows, your body will burn more calories than normal, and there is no risk of entering starvation mode.

It is important that you stick with the fast that you chose and don't go overboard with this. If you don't eat healthy foods during your eating window, or you choose to eat too few calories during that time, and your fasts are too long, you could risk entering starvation mode and dealing with all the issues that come with that. However, if you follow your chosen intermittent fast well and you eat the right foods, you don't have to worry about this issue.

Who Would Benefit the Most from Intermittent Fasting?

Almost everyone can benefit from going on an intermittent fast. It helps to speed up the metabolism, can give you more energy, puts the body in fat burning mode and often can result in weight loss and health benefits, unlike any other diet plan. People who would benefit the most from starting an intermittent fast are:

- Those who want to lose weight.

- Those who want to change their eating habits.

- Weightlifters and bodybuilders.

•Those who want to learn how to listen to their bodies more and learn when they are hungry, thirsty, or need to deal with something.

•Those who want to make life easier with fewer meals to plan.

•Those who want to improve their heart health.

•Those who want to help fight off diabetes.

•Those who are looking to keep the brain strong and working well.

•Those who are interested in getting rid of belly fat.

Is There Anyone Who Shouldn't Go on an Intermittent Fast?

While an intermittent fast can be a great way to help improve your health and lose weight, some individuals should consider not doing an intermittent fast. These individuals may experience trouble getting the right amount of nutrition through the day when they fast, and they may have to worry about medications or other issues that fasting can aggravate. People who should consider not doing an intermittent fast, or at least should discuss it with their doctor ahead of time, include:

•Children and teenagers who are still developing and growing.

•Women who are currently pregnant.

•Women who are currently breastfeeding.

•People who have recently had surgery and are recovering.

•People with certain eating disorders.

•Those who are currently underweight.

•Those who are dealing with diabetes that is controlled with insulin.

•Some types of medications can be negatively affected by an intermittent fast as well. Make sure to discuss this with your doctor before starting.

Intermittent fasting is a great eating plan that makes it easy for you to lose weight and improve your health. However, concerning the above conditions, it can be a challenge to fast regarding getting adequate nutrition throughout the day, and not just during short eating windows.

Chapter 2: How Does Intermittent Fasting Help Burn Fat and Weight Loss?

When you go on an intermittent fast, you force the body to stop relying on a constant source of glucose to fuel it. Since you go so long without eating, your body still has to look for some form of fuel to help it function and do well. It will resort to burning the stored glycogen of the body, or the stored body fat. Just by doing these short-term fasts each day, you will burn through the extra fat on your body, cut out calories, and lose weight faster than ever before.

Intermittent fasting is all about adding short fasts into your daily life. The goal is to reduce the number of calories that you consume and increase how fast the metabolism runs at the same time. This can result in not only a bunch of great health benefits but also some weight loss as well. But why is intermittent fasting so effective at helping you to burn fat and lose weight? Let's look at some of the ways that intermittent fasting will affect your body and help you get the results that you want.

Intermittent Fasting and How It Affects Your Hormones

The body fat that you carry around is simply just the way that the body stores any unused energy or calories that you take in. When you go through a period of not eating anything, your body is going to experience changes that can help you access your stored energy better. This can be the changes in your hormones and the activity of your nervous system.

During the fast, you will notice that there are a few changes that occur in your metabolism including:

>•Norepinephrine: The nervous system is going to send this hormone to your stored fat cells. This hormone causes the fat cells to break down into free fatty acids. The body can then take these fatty acids and use them as energy.

>•HGH or human growth hormone: Levels of the hormone can increase like crazy. This hormone can help aid in many processes of the body, including muscle gain and fat loss.

>•Insulin: When you eat any food, your insulin is going to increase. But when you go on a fast, your insulin levels will decrease quite a bit. Lower levels of insulin in the body will help you burn more fat.

Despite what proponents of five to six meals each day say, going on these short-term fasts can actually help you increase the amount of fat that you burn during the day. In fact, two studies found that fasting for a 48-hour time period can help boost your metabolism by up to 14 percent.

The amazing thing about intermittent fasting is that it helps you to affect your hormones in a natural way. As long as your fasting period doesn't last for more than 48 hours, you are not going to cause any negative harm to the body. Instead, you will positively affect your hormones, so they behave in a way that is beneficial to you. You will be better able to regulate your insulin levels, keep your metabolism moving fast, and even help you to feel less hungry throughout the day.

However, you need to be careful with this one. If you go for a period that is too long, such as a 72-hour fast, you can actually suppress your metabolism. Stick with these shorter-term fasts to get the most benefits and the faster metabolism from fasting.

Fasting Is a Great Way to Reduce Your Calories and Lose Weight Naturally

The main reason that intermittent fasts work to help you lose weight is because they make it easier for you to eat fewer calories without feeling deprived. All the protocols for fasting involve skipping meals. Unless you go crazy with compensating for your calories during the eating period, you can take in fewer calories during the day.

According to a review study that was done in 2014, intermittent fasting reduced the body weight of participants by up to 8 percent over a time period that lasted between three to 24 weeks. When looking at this rapid weight loss rate, people were able to lose about 0.55 pounds each week when doing intermittent fasting, but about 1.65 pounds each week when they went on an alternate fasting diet. Those who were in this review also showed that people lost between four to seven percent of their waist circumference, which showed that they also lost belly fat during this time.

These results are impressive and show that alternate day fasting and intermittent fasting can be useful when it comes to losing weight. In addition, the benefits of fasting can go beyond weight loss. It has many benefits on the health of your metabolism and can help expand your lifespan, prevent chronic diseases, and so much more.

While intermittent fasting often doesn't require calorie counting because you can naturally reduce your calories with this method, you may still want to watch your total calories and the types of food that you are eating. Studies have shown that continuous calorie restriction and intermittent fasting have the same results when it comes to weight loss, but intermittent fasting is often seen as much easier to follow.

While some preliminary studies show that intermittent fasting and continuous calorie restriction will give about the same results when it comes to calories burnt and weight loss, many people find that sticking with the intermittent fast is easier. Moreover, when an eating plan is more effective to stick with, people are more likely to follow it and see results.

Intermittent Fasting Can Help You Keep Your Muscle Tone When You Diet

One thing that can happen when you go on a diet is that the body may burn through some of the muscle as well as the fat. However, there are a few studies that show how intermittent fasting can be beneficial to helping you hold onto your muscle, even while you are losing body fat.

With one review study, it was found that doing calorie restriction through intermittent fasting can cause a similar amount of weight loss as continuous calorie restriction. However, one difference is that the former resulted in a smaller reduction in muscle mass through that time.

In the study that looked at calorie restriction, there was about 25 percent of the weight loss that was a result of lost muscle mass. But with intermittent fasting, the amount of weight that was lost to reduced muscle mass was only ten percent. In one of the studies, those who participated would eat the same number of calories as before, but they would just have one large meal in the evening rather than having the calories spread out throughout the day. These participants ended up losing body fat while increasing their muscle mass compared to regular dieting. There were also a ton of other beneficial changes to the health markers in those who did this kind of intermittent fasting.

Intermittent Fasting Not Only Helps with Weight Loss but Also with Making Healthy Eating Easier

One of the best benefits that come with intermittent fasting, in addition to the weight loss and all the health benefits, is that this eating plan is really simple. There are many methods that you can choose to go with; however, all of them are simple and don't contain a lot of hard to follow rules. Simply stick with the eating and fasting windows that are listed in your protocol, and you are going to see some great results.

Compared to some of the other diet plans that you may have tried out in the past, intermittent fasting is going to be simple and easy. You eat at certain times, you avoid eating at others, and you fill your body with lots of healthy nutrients when you can. If you can follow these rules, you will see all the results that you need from intermittent fasting.

Compared to other dieting plans that you can choose, intermittent fasting can provide you with the best results. It naturally works with your body to help you burn fat fast and speeds up your metabolism, so you can burn more calories and lose weight. Add to all this the simplicity of it. It is no wonder that many people choose to go with this eating plan rather than sticking with one of their old dieting plans.

Chapter 3: The Art of Autophagy: How Intermittent Fasting Can Help Clean out the Body

One neat thing that can happen when you are on an intermittent fast is a process that is known as autophagy. This word derives from the Greek word *auto*, which means 'self', and *phagein*, which means 'to eat'. So, if we are looking at the literal meaning of the word, we are looking at a word that means to eat oneself. Of course, this is not exactly what we mean by autophagy.

Instead, we mean that we are looking at the mechanism of the body to get rid of any waste, any old cells, or anything that has broken down once the body doesn't have enough energy to sustain it. It is regulated and orderly and helps the body to stay healthy and not hold onto all the waste that the body releases through your daily life.

Autophagy was first heard about in 1962 when researchers noted that the number of lysosomes in rat liver cells after there was an infusion of glucagon ended up increasing. The lysosomes are the part of the cell that is responsible for destroying stuff. This process was eventually coined as autophagy. The damaged subcellular parts, as well as any unused proteins in the cells, were marked for destruction and then sent over to the lysosomes to help finish up the job.

One of the parts that are important for regulating autophagy is the kinase that goes by the name of mTOR or the mammalian target of rapamycin. When this is activated, it suppresses the process of autophagy. However, when this regulator is dormant, the process of autophagy is promoted and works better.

What Will Activate the Process of Autophagy?

The biggest thing that can activate autophagy is nutrient deprivation. Remember that glucagon is pretty much the opposite of insulin. If the levels of insulin in the body go up, then glucagon is going to go down. The opposite can also be true. If insulin levels go down, then the levels of glucagon will go up. Any time that we eat something, our levels of insulin are going to go up, and it makes it hard for the glucagon because it goes down. If glucagon doesn't have time to elevate at all because you are eating all day long, then you won't be able to have the process of autophagy in the body. Fasting can raise glucagon, which means it is one of the best ways to boost autophagy.

This is the basics of cellular cleansing. The body is going to identify the old and bad cellular equipment in the body and will put a little mark on it for destruction. If all this junk stays in the body and isn't cleaned out, it often affects the aging process in the body.

Not only can fasting help to stimulate this autophagy process, but it can also help in other ways as well. When you fast and stimulate autophagy, you are cleaning out all the old proteins and parts of the cells. In addition, fasting can also stimulate a growth hormone. This hormone will tell the body to start producing the new replacement parts in the body. So, when you go on one of these fasts, you are effectively giving your body a new renovation.

You have to take the time to get rid of all the old stuff before you have a chance to put in any of the new. Think about doing a renovation in your kitchen. If you have an older kitchen that is an eyesore, you must go through it and get rid of all the old cabinets and countertops and everything else to make room for the new stuff. This same idea is important when it comes to the building up of cells in the body. If you just try to build up new cells in the body, without removing all the bad stuff first, it is just going to end up a mess.

Intermittent fasting can really help to handle this. It ensures that you can take care of the body, remove all the old stuff that is there, and then make room for the new. Fasting can provide a natural detox that can improve your health and reverse the aging process, and it is so simple to follow.

A Process That Is Highly Controlled

The process of autophagy is very regulated. If it was able to run out of control, it could be very detrimental to the body, so it is controlled. In the mammalian cells, total depletion of amino acids can be a very strong signal for this process to control, but the role of the individual amino acids can be more variable. On the other hand, the amino acid of the plasma will vary only a little bit. The insulin signals, the growth factor signals, and the amino acid signals are going to converge on the mTOR pathway and will all work to regulate this process.

During autophagy, you can naturally clean out the body. This provides a natural detox that is so good when it comes to your health and weight loss. In a traditional American diet, though, it is very hard to go on a fast. Remember, autophagy can't happen when insulin levels are high. And insulin levels are going to be high if you are constantly eating all the time.

A typical American has a diet that allows them to eat something from the moment they get up until the moment they go to sleep. This makes it hard to let the process of autophagy even start and can cause aging, cancer, Alzheimer's, and other issues.

When you spend time on a fast, you will see that things change. Your levels of insulin will go down, allowing glucagon to increase and the process of autophagy to occur. You have to give your body some time to see this change though. The fast doesn't have to be long, but either a full day fast once or twice a week or a short daily fast can be enough to help you clean out the body, while also creating new cells and giving them room to grow at the same time.

Chapter 4: The Different Types of Fasts That You Can Go On

When we talk about intermittent fasting, there are a few different options that you can consider. Some involve doing a small fast each day while others are full-day fasts during the week. Some of these options are:

The 16/8 Method

This popular method requires a small fast daily that lasts about 16 hours. During that time, you are not allowed to eat any solid food. Options like coffee, water, and other non-caloric beverages can be consumed to help keep you full and ensure that you stay hydrated. After the fast is done, you are given an eight-hour window to eat.

This method is pretty easy to follow. It is as simple as finishing dinner one night and then waiting until lunchtime to eat your next meal. If you get up in the morning, get the kids off to school and do some work, the morning will fly by, and soon it will be time to eat. You can do other variations as well as having an early dinner, so you can eat breakfast, as long as you stay in that eight-hour eating window.

There are also different options that you can choose with this method. Some people need a longer eating window to start out, so they may fast for 14 to 15 hours, and then have their eating window for the remaining hours. No matter how you do it, make sure that your eating window is full of lots of healthy and delicious foods, ones that will keep you full, keep those cravings away, and help you lose weight.

Eat Stop Eat

This method has you pick one to two days during the week where you will do a 24-hour fast. During this time, you are not allowed to eat anything solid. You can enjoy beverages, especially water, non-caloric beverages, and coffee. You have to wait until the fast is over before you can eat anything else. For the other days of the week, you can eat normally, and as healthy as possible.

This method doesn't need to be as complicated as it sounds. You don't have to go from supper one day, miss a meal the next day, and then finally have breakfast two days later. This is technically a 36-hour fast. So instead, you can go from supper one night and then eat the next day at supper. Or you can go from lunch one day to lunch the second, or even breakfast to breakfast. Many people who do the 'eat stop eat' method will go from supper to supper because this helps them to never go to bed hungry.

The 5:2 Diet

This method works like alternate day fasting, but you only go on a fast for two days out of the week. You can pick any two days that you want; just make sure they are not consecutive. During those fasting days, you need to keep your calorie count to 500 or less for the entire day.

There are a few options here. You can choose to take that 500 calories and split it up into two meals. This allows you to still get some food in throughout the day and is sometimes easier for you to accomplish. Others find that when they are fasting, once they start eating, it is hard to stop, and they need to eat more than 250 calories for that meal. These individuals may find that saving the calories and eating all 500 at once is better. They can save the calories for supper, staying in the fast a bit longer, and then splurge a bit more when they finally do get to eat that day.

For the other five days of the week, you can eat normally. Try to stick with a healthy diet with lots of the nutrients the body needs. When you combine a few days a week with only 500 calories and then eat normally during the normal days, you can still end up with a deficit at the end of the week.

The Warrior Diet

The warrior diet follows the same idea as the 16/8 method but takes things a little bit further with a shorter eating window. This diet was originally developed to help weightlifters and bodybuilders burn through any excess body fat and get stronger for competitions, but this doesn't mean that anyone can't give it a try to help lose weight and feel better.

The warrior diet puts the individual on a schedule where they fast for 20 hours during the day. During this time, you can have a few fresh fruits and vegetables, as long as you consume them raw, and you only eat a few hundred calories or less worth of those each day. You should not be getting a ton of calories from this grazing before your eating window. This is only meant to help quell your eating patterns a bit.

For the other four hours of the day, you are allowed to eat. You can choose to split that time up into two meals, or you can have just one big meal to end your day. You need to make sure that you get in all the nutrients that the body needs during this time. Since you are limiting your eating window so much, it is easier to feel full on fewer calories, and your body can spend most of the day in fat burning mode.

The warrior diet is often hard to get started on, especially if you are used to eating all day long and providing your body with a constant supply of glucose. It is a long time to go without eating, and then you have to choose good foods, to provide your body with enough nutrition, which can be difficult. You may want to start with one of the other fasting methods like the 16/8 method to make it easier to start.

The Master Cleanse

The Master Cleanse is usually considered as too restrictive and too long of a fast to fit under the idea of intermittent fasting, but we are going to look at it to see how it is different from intermittent fasting.

The Master Cleanse has gained popularity in the past few years due to many celebrities who have claimed to go on it to lose a lot of weight. The ideas behind this kind of cleanse are often not very healthy, and while you will probably lose a lot of weight, much of it will come back as soon as you start to eat a healthy diet again.

This diet is also called The Lemonade Diet, and it is a liquid only fast. The claim with this fast is that if you stick with it for ten days or so, you will drop weight, clean out your system, and feel more energetic and healthier. It also states that this cleanse can help you curb cravings for unhealthy foods.

During the fast, you can only drink a herbal laxative tea, lemonade, and then a salt water drink for ten days. After the ten days are up, it is fine to add some foods back in slowly, but you will need to take it slowly. Your body has been on low calories for more than a week so bombarding it with a ton of calories is never a good idea. Start the first few days with some soups and a little juice and then move to fresh produce. Slowly move up until you are back to a healthy diet plan.

Since you are taking in fewer calories than before, it's likely that this fast will help you lose weight. However, the ingredients that you can have on this fast are going to be so low in calories that you could lose water weight, muscle tone, and more. And since you are not going to be able to stay on this diet plan forever, it is likely that when you add more calories back into your diet, the weight will come back.

The Master Cleanse is hard and may cause unneeded stress on your digestive system and hormones. It is often better to go with one of the shorter fasts mentioned earlier because they can provide you with all the health benefits that you need without causing harm to your body. If you are worried about getting on a fast and fighting off those cravings, a version of the Master Cleanse can be helpful, but consider doing it for just a few days, rather than ten.

Chapter 5: What Is the Difference Between Intermittent Fasting, Alternate Day Fasting, and Extended Fasting?

As you look at the world of fasting and do some research, you may notice that there are actually many kinds of fasts. Some of these are intermittent fasting methods, but others are unique, and you may wonder how they compare to intermittent fasting. Let's take a look at the difference between intermittent fasting, alternate day fasting, and extended fasting and the benefits and negatives of following each type of fasting.

Intermittent Fasting

This is simple to follow, and there are a few different methods that you can pick from to suit your needs. An intermittent fast requires you to split up your day between eating times and fasting times. The goal is to make your fasting time longer than your eating times. This gives the body time to get into a fasting state, encouraging autophagy and making it easier for you to burn the fat stored in your body.

There are a few different types of intermittent fasting. Some people will spend one or two days a week fasting for a whole day, or do a smaller fast every day of the week, or, like the alternate day fasting (described below), fast three or four days of the week.

All these methods can be effective, and it often depends on the method that works the best for your schedule. These fasts all allow you to take a break from eating all the time, so your insulin levels can stabilize and the natural fat burning and cleaning out process of the body can occur.

The nice thing about intermittent fasting is that it can naturally fit into your current schedule and it doesn't necessarily consist of doing much work. In addition, the fast is short enough that you can get all the health and weight loss benefits without having to worry about entering starvation mode and all the problems that can entail.

Alternate Day Fasting

Alternate day fasting is one of the options that you can choose to help you with intermittent fasting. This method involves fasting every other day of the week. The other days can be regular eating days, and you can enjoy whatever you would like. The most common version of this diet is similar to the 5:2 diet. With this modified version, which can be a bit easier for some people to follow, you are allowed to have 500 calories on your fasting days.

When you see a study done on intermittent fasting, it is most likely to have been done on the alternate day fasting. This type of fasting can be a powerful way to lose some weight while also reducing some of the risks you have for heart disease and can prevent type 2 diabetes.

The basic idea that comes with this type of fast is that you are going to fast on one day, then eat normally on the second. Then you will alternate back and forth between the regular diet days and the fasting days. This means that you only need to place restrictions on what you are eating half the time. During your fasting days, you can drink as much water and other calorie-free beverages as you need to keep yourself hydrated.

If you are following this method, there is an option to modify it if you find it too hard not to eat anything that many days of the week. You can consume up to 500 calories during your fasting days. This still gives you a calorie deficit since it is much less than what you need during the whole week. The benefits that you get with this are going to be similar, regardless of whether you have the calories placed at dinner, lunch, or split up through the day.

While this may seem like an extreme version of intermittent fasting, one that is going to be difficult to do, studies have shown that many people like alternate day fasting and find it easier to stick with compared to regular calorie restriction. Moreover, most of the studies on this kind of fasting focus on the modified version so this can make things even easier.

Extended Fasting

Long-term fasting can often take different forms. The most extreme of these is a dry fast where you don't drink any food or water, but this is often not advisable because not only are you missing out on food, but you are missing out on some of the hydration that you need. There is also a water fast, which means that you can have all the water and hydration that you need, but you won't consume any calories during the fast. Some people may go on a juice fast or even a low-calorie protein fast.

These extended fasts are going to last longer than the other two types of fasts. Alternate day fasting is every other day and can be a form of intermittent fasting. Intermittent fasting is usually 24 hours or less and can either happen a few days a week, every other day of the week, or every day of the week for certain hours. However, with extended fasting, you are going to spend even longer fasting. Often, people will spend a week or more on one of these fasts.

We are going to look at one of the most common extended fasts that you can choose. This one is a water fast and is often done for extreme weight loss quickly or for religious purposes. We will look at the benefits, the negatives, and some of the precautions.

The biggest reason that someone will choose to go on an extended fast is to help with weight loss. If you don't eat anything for an extended period, your body will drop the weight. For the first day of the fast, you are going to see the body use up all the glycogen that is in the liver. Then the body will rely on what it has stored, either fat or protein.

After you get through this first day or so, your body may lose about one to two pounds each day. This comes from using up the protein in the body and shedding some water weight. The body will decide that burning muscle is not a good thing since you need your heart to pump to keep you alive and will work on burning through the stored fat. Since fat is more energy dense for each pound compared to protein, the weight loss may slow down after the first few days. It is still rapid weight loss, though, and can result in one pound every two days.

The problem with this is that once you go back to your old ways of eating, you are most likely to gain all the weight, or at least most of it, back. And there are sometimes dangerous consequences to this kind of fasting. Even a fast that is less than a few weeks can cause issues. This extreme type of fasting can put two stress types on the heart. First, it is going to cannibalize the muscles of the heart to use for fuel. The body is going to try to conserve muscle during a fast, but sometimes it has to sacrifice it to keep you alive, and this can affect the heart.

In addition, strict water fasting can put you at a higher risk for heart failure because when you are on one of these fasts, the intracellular stores of minerals that protect the heart are going to be depleted. This could cause mineral deprivation and can be tragic. In addition, if you get sick during this time, it is harder to fight illness and can put you at risk as well.

Some people who go on very extreme extended fasts may see even more serious effects, and some have even died. This is not very common, and the biggest case of this happening was in 1981 when ten political prisoners went on a fast for 46 to 73 days and starved themselves to death during a hunger strike.

An extended fast can be useful in some cases: it can help you to lose a lot of weight quickly; put the body into ketosis, so it starts to burn off some of the excess fat that is hanging around the body; and, in some cases, helps the individual develop a healthier relationship with food that they can carry forward into the future. However, before you go on one of these fasts, you must make sure you are in good health. Talk it over with your doctor to make sure you are being safe, and make sure that you don't go on an extended fast that is too long.

Chapter 6: Intermittent Fasting and Improved Insulin Sensitivity

Now it is time to move onto some of the benefits that you can get when you decide to implement an intermittent fast. First, we will look at how intermittent fasting can help improve your insulin levels. Insulin is a hormone that the pancreas will produce, and it can play a vital role in helping the body regulate and control your levels of blood sugar. Insulin can be helpful in making sure your blood sugars never go too low or too high.

Despite the bad reputation of insulin, your body does need it to function. The body is going to use sugar, also known as glucose, to function and it gets this from the food you eat. However, the body can't directly absorb this nutrient, and it needs some help. The beta cells that are found in the pancreas will release insulin into your bloodstream to help the sugar get absorbed by the cells and be used as a form of energy. Without this insulin, sugar can't be absorbed properly and will just sit around.

If the body receives more sugar that it needs, insulin will take that sugar and store it in the liver to use later when you need some extra, such as when you are fasting or exercising. Insulin has another job of letting the liver know when it should stop releasing glucose into the blood.

In some cases, the body will not be able to produce enough insulin. Or there could be the problem of insulin having a minimal effect on the cells of the body. When this happens, your levels of blood sugar may get too high. This is a condition that is known as hyperglycemia. This condition can cause many other complications to your health, including loss of consciousness, vomiting, infections, numbness, weight loss, tiredness, hunger, thirst, and frequent trips to the bathroom.

What Does Insulin Resistance Mean?

Insulin resistance is going to occur whenever the cells in your body won't respond to insulin properly and aren't able to absorb the glucose that is in the blood. This is going to force the pancreas to get to work and produce more of the insulin that you need. In some cases, this may get severe enough that you will need to take injections of insulin. This extra insulin is meant to help the cells of the body absorb the glucose that you eat. This issue is a common occurrence in those with type 2 diabetes and prediabetes.

Certain individuals are more likely to suffer from either prediabetes or type 2 diabetes where the body's cells just don't respond to the insulin that is there. When this happens, it can mean that a lot of extra glucose is hanging around in the blood and storing that extra nutrient as body fat. People who might be at a higher risk for these conditions include:

- Those who are on some types of medications, such as HIV medications and antipsychotics.

- Those who suffer from various sleep conditions like sleep apnea.

•Those who are Hispanic, American Indian, Asian American, and African American.

•Those who have had issues with their heart health or who suffered from a stroke in the past.

•Those who have poor levels of cholesterol and high blood pressure.

•Those who don't get enough physical activity into their day.

•Those who already have a family member who suffers from diabetes.

•Those who are 45 years or older.

•Those who are obese or overweight.

There is still research being done on the exact cause of this insulin resistance. However, it is believed that lack of activity and excess weight are the two main factors that can cause this. Helping yourself keep at a healthy weight and making sure that you get up and be active on a regular basis may be the key to preventing this insulin resistance.

How Will an Intermittent Fast Affect My Insulin Levels?

You will quickly find that intermittent fasting can do a great deal of good when it comes to increasing your lipolysis and lowering your levels of insulin. Lipolysis is a process of the fat cells breaking down in the body. When you fast for a longer period, it can reduce the deposits of fat that are in your body. As these deposits get smaller, the cells in the liver and the muscles start to respond more to the insulin that is there.

This can make it so much easier for the insulin and glucose in the body to move into the cells and can decrease your risk of high blood sugar. It can also be good for the cells as well.

When you have lots of food readily available, the body is going to be less sensitive to insulin. The higher insulin levels that are produced to compensate for this will inhibit the secretion of HGH. In fact, HGH and insulin are going to work in opposing manners. The main role of insulin is to focus on storing energy and pro-inflammatory functions while HGH focuses on optimizing the use of fuel, tissue repair, and stopping inflammation.

When your insulin levels are higher, the HGH levels will be lower. Studies show that elevated insulin levels can help diminish the neuronal autophagy that we talked about earlier. When your body can't go through the process of autophagy, old and damaged cells are going to stick around, and the body will run into trouble functioning the right way.

When the body goes on a fast, it can help to reduce those levels of insulin. The body isn't receiving food, and insulin is only released when there is food that can be turned into glucose and used as energy by the body. Without food, the body won't produce insulin, and the levels go down.

With the traditional way of eating, we often feed the body nonstop, causing our insulin levels to be high. The cells become less sensitive to the insulin because they are bombarded with it all the time. In addition, the higher insulin levels can cause trouble with autophagy occurring and leads to an increase in old and damaged cells in the body.

Fasting can help solve this issue. It turns off insulin production during parts of the day, allowing the cells to have a break. When the cells aren't as bombarded with insulin, it can increase their sensitivity to it later. They will, over time, be better able to absorb the nutrients that you take in due to this change in sensitivity, which is exactly what you want when it comes to preventing or reversing diabetes. You also give the body a chance to lower insulin levels so that autophagy can occur and clean out the body.

If you simply continue to eat nonstop, you are making the problem worse. Insulin will continue to rise, and you will continue to see a reduction in the sensitivity of your cells to insulin. This is how prediabetes and type 2 diabetes end up occurring. Fasting can help give your body a break, to reduce your levels of insulin, so you can see better results with reducing your risk of diabetes.

How Long Do I Need to Do a Fast to Reduce My Levels of Insulin?

Your levels of insulin are going to rise any time you eat. However, the amount that these levels rise will depend on what you eat. The more carbs you take in, the higher your insulin levels and the more likely that sensitivity in the cells will be reduced. These higher insulin levels can easily stay high for a few hours after you eat, and then after you go some time without eating, they will slowly start to fall again.

According to Intensive Dietary Management, your insulin levels will start falling sometime between six to 24 hours after you start fasting as your glycogen starts to get broken down and is used by the body as a source of energy. This phase is going to be known as the post-absorptive phase. After 24 to 48 hours, the body is going to switch over and will enter the gluconeogenesis state.

During this state, the liver is going to take amino acids and start producing new glucose. Then, after 48 to 72 hours of fasting, the body will enter a process of ketosis. This is when your insulin levels will start to really fall low, and the body will turn to fat as its energy source. Through this process, you will see that the easiest way for you to reduce the levels of insulin in your body is to go on a fast and not eat.

Dr. Naiman, who is known for running the Burn Fat Not Sugar website, argues that fasting between 18 to 24 hours is the best because insulin levels are going to see the biggest drop off during this time while you still see the fat breakdown, or lipolysis, increase. However, it appears that going on a fast for a longer period, such as for 24 hours, could have the biggest effect when it comes to reducing your insulin levels.

Therefore, alternate day fasting is so popular. There are many studies out there that show how alternate day fasting can help decrease fat, body weight, and insulin. In one of these studies, published in the US National Library of Medicine, 16 participants, eight women, and eight men, who weren't obese at the start of the study, went on an alternate day fasting schedule for a period of 22 days. During this time, the researchers looked at various numbers to help them see what occurred during the fast, including the resting metabolic rate, body composition, weight, insulin, ghrelin, and fasting serum glucose to name a few items.

The results showed many interesting things. First, most of the subjects lost an average of 2.5 percent of their initial body weight and their insulin levels decreased by 57 percent, plus or minus four percent on average. However, some scores didn't change up, including ghrelin, glucose, and RMR. Hunger didn't seem to decrease on any of the fasting days which showed that some of the participants might run into difficulties if they continued this diet over the long term. To keep this diet going over the long term, it may be best to do the modified version of alternate day fasting to help add in a meal on that fasting day.

Another case study, found in the Journal of Insulin Resistance, followed a patient with type 2 diabetes from Ontario for four months. At the beginning of the study, the patient was fasting for 24 hours three times a week. However, over the course of the study, that patient started to increase their fasting sessions to 42 hours two or three times each week.

When this study was done, the patient had lost 17.8 percent of their body weight, and their waist was 11 percent smaller. However, what was the most surprising effect of this change was that the patient was able to discontinue using insulin treatments at the end of the fast, despite having been on insulin for more than ten years prior.

Although these are small studies, they give a good idea on how effective fasting can be at reducing your levels of insulin and helping you to reduce your risks of developing diabetes in the future. It can even help optimize the levels of insulin in those who already have type 2 diabetes and who are trying to properly manage it for their health. While these results may not be the same for everyone who goes on an intermittent fast, they still provide some insight into how great this eating plan can be.

Chapter 7: Intermittent Fasting and Reduced Levels of Inflammation Throughout the Body

Inflammation is not always a bad thing. It is often the start of the healing process inside the body. While many people strive to reduce inflammation after they suffer an injury, some inflammation, if it is minimal and doesn't stick around for a long time, can be beneficial because it tells the body that it is time to start healing. However, when inflammation is constantly around, or it lasts longer than normal, major health problems can occur.

Inflammation can become a bad thing when it sticks around, and it is going to play a big role in many chronic conditions like cancer, asthma, obesity, and Crohn's disease. Chronic inflammation can be problematic because it can be the start of other issues like back pain, osteoporosis, and arthritis. Add to all this the growing proof that inflammation can cause other issues, such as Alzheimer's, obesity, dementia, and depression. It is no wonder that many people are afraid of inflammation.

There are many different reasons that you may suffer from inflammation, but often it is caused by poor lifestyle choices. It could be from consuming too much processed foods and sugars or not getting enough physical activity in your life. Other issues that could cause this inflammation include gut health problems, exhaustion, and stress.

Is It Possible for Intermittent Fasting to Reduce Inflammation?

There is some evidence that shows how intermittent fasting can be a very effective way to reduce inflammation throughout the body. Research shows how intermittent fasting could have a protective effect against several issues, including inflammation, high insulin levels, and high blood pressure. Intermittent fasting could also help with conditions that increase inflammation, including autoimmune conditions and type 2 diabetes.

In one of these studies, the researcher would feed mice either a high-fat or low-fat diet for a period of ten to 12 weeks. After fasting, the mice who were fed a low-fat diet lost more body weight compared to the other group, did better on learning tasks and memory, and showed more locomotor activity. The mice who were on the low-fat diet also had an improved immune and nervous system function. The conclusion here is that fasting has an anti-inflammatory effect on our bodies, which is something that the high-fat diet may prevent from happening.

Another study looked at those who went on a Ramadan fast. This study was done in 2017 and published in the US National Library of Medicine. It compared 83 people with NAFLD or nonalcoholic fatty liver disease. 42 of these individuals fasted and 41 were the control group who didn't fast. Those who fasted had big reductions in inflammation, insulin resistance, plasma insulin, and glucose compared to the other group.

How Can Intermittent Fasting Help Reduce Inflammation?

There are many ways that intermittent fasting can help reduce inflammation throughout the body. Some of these include:

- Promotes autophagy: We have discussed this briefly, but when the process of autophagy is allowed to occur, the inflammation in the body will go down as it cleans itself out.

- Promotes BHB: Beta-hydroxybutyrate is one of the three main types of ketones that the mitochondria of the liver produce. This one can protect the body against inflammation, improve cognition, can reduce the risk of cancer, and regulates appetite. There are several times when the body is going to produce BHB including:

  - When you severely restrict your calories, or you go on a fast.

  - You perform high-intensity exercises.

  - You consume a supplement that has BHB inside it.

  - You consume a salt, such as calcium or magnesium, that can be absorbed easily in the body.

  - You follow a ketogenic diet or one that is high fat and low carb.

- Improves your sensitivity to insulin: When the cells are sensitive to the insulin that you produce, they will easily absorb the glucose that is in your food. However, when the sensitivity goes down, or you eat too much of the glucose-producing foods, the cells won't take it up. This glucose sits around the body and can cause a lot of inflammation. Intermittent fasting can help to kick up the sensitivity of the cells to insulin, so they can absorb the glucose and not deal with all the inflammation inside.

•Lowers Leukotriene B4 (LTB4): LTB4 is a proinflammatory lipid that is going to increase inflammation quite a bit. It can play a role in chronic inflammation and can be responsible for many different health conditions, including inflammatory bowel disease, asthma, and rheumatoid arthritis. Research shows that LTB4 can also cause resistance to insulin in mice. Fasting is one way to lower the levels of LTB4 in the body to help reduce some of the inflammation.

•Fights off oxidative stress: This kind of stress occurs when there is a big imbalance between the antioxidants and free radicals in the body. The free radicals are unstable molecules that will oxidize with the other molecules found in your body. This can result in damage to tissues, DNA, and cells and can lead to many inflammatory conditions. These free radicals can be caused by things like:

    oEating too many carbs, sugars, and calories. The body must convert these into energy, and it takes a lot of work. This can lead to more of the free radicals through the body.

    oNot getting enough exercise. You need to keep your body in optimal shape to boost your immunity and fight off the oxidative stress.

    oAlcohol consumption has been shown to increase inflammation.

    oCigarettes contain many bad chemicals that can increase the risk of oxidative stress.

    oChronic stress has been shown to have a huge negative impact on your overall health, and if it happens often, it can lead to inflammation.

oVarious environmental factors. This could include radiation, ozone, and pollution.

What Does the Research Have to Say About All This?

There has been a lot of research done on intermittent fasting, and some of it shows how fasting could help to protect you against inflammation and oxidative stress in the body. One of these studies looked at alternate day fasting and its effects on overweight adults who were suffering from asthma. Ten of the patients were put on a diet where they would fast every other day, or do an alternate day fast, for eight weeks. At the end of this study, those patients showed a huge reduction in the amount of inflammation they had.

In another clinical trial, researchers decided to look at how fasting would be able to change the cells in the body. 24 participants were invited, and they were to practice intermittent fasting for two three-week sessions. During the first of the three-week sessions, the participants went on what was considered a modified intermittent fasting diet. On this, they would alternate between fasting days where they took in 25 percent of their normal caloric intake and feasting days where they would take in 75 percent of their normal calories.

For the second of the three-week sessions, the participants followed that same kind of modified fasting diet, but then they also took some supplements, including an anti-oxidant, vitamin E, and vitamin A.

What the researchers were trying to find out is if fasting would improve oxidative stress and if the stress would produce cells that were stronger in these participants. The researchers also wanted to know if taking any antioxidants would inhibit the cells from getting any stronger because those antioxidants could potentially shelter the cells from oxidative stress and from free radicals in the body.

What the researchers found was that fasting was able to help produce more SIRT3, a gene that is going to help improve cells and can inhibit the production of free radicals. Participants in this study also ended up with lower levels of insulin, which helped protect them against developing diabetes.

One thing that was interesting about this study is that taking vitamin E and C seemed to negate some of the positive benefits the participants had when they went on a fast. The belief here is that these antioxidants sheltered the cells from any oxidative stress. Because of this, the cells couldn't develop any defense mechanisms and become stronger to help them deal with any type of stressful stimuli. If you are using intermittent fasting to help prevent inflammation in the body, it is best just to use that and not add in any supplements or antioxidants – since these seem to protect the cells and makes it hard for them to become any stronger.

As you can see, intermittent fasting can be an effective way to help you reduce inflammation and oxidative stress in the body. It is simple to follow, helps you to reduce many issues that can cause inflammation, and can help you finally get some relief!

Chapter 8: Lowering Triglyceride and Cholesterol Levels

Cholesterol is made up of proteins and fat, or lipids, that produce hormones and help your body to break down fats. Cholesterol has gotten kind of a bad name, but it is something that is needed to help keep the body healthy. However, if you have too much cholesterol, it could cause fatty deposits to build up in your blood vessels. This could increase the risk of cardiovascular problems, including coronary artery disease, stroke, and heart attack.

The levels of your cholesterol will be determined by your diet and your genetics. Most cholesterol is going to be produced in the liver, but then you can also get plenty of it from the foods that you consume. Eating foods that have high levels of trans fat, saturated fats, and cholesterol can make your levels of cholesterol increase. Certain foods naturally have more cholesterol in them, so it is important to watch out for them.

High levels of cholesterol can cause atherosclerosis and health complications. Atherosclerosis is a process that will cause plaque to build up in your blood vessels. This can end up narrowing down the blood vessels and will increase your risks of a stroke and heart attack. In fact, heart disease and heart attacks are one of the leading causes of death in the world. Therefore, it is so important to monitor your cholesterol levels as much as possible.

You also need to watch out for your triglyceride levels. Triglycerides are a type of fat that is found in the body because the body can convert some of the food that you eat into this fat. The body will either use these as energy, or it will store them up in the fat cells to use later. If you store too much of this, it can cause fat to accumulate in the body.

These triglycerides are going to be composed of polyunsaturated, monounsaturated, and saturated fats. Each of these types of fat can create a foundation of monounsaturated fatty acids, polyunsaturated fatty acids, and saturated fats. Since these are a type of fat, they are going to get converted into glycerol and free fatty acids any time that you fast, and then they are used as energy. In comparison, cholesterol, during the fast, will be converted to make certain types of hormones or to repair cells.

Your levels of triglycerides can give you a good indication of what you have eaten recently, but the cholesterol is going to give you an idea of what you have consumed over a long period of time. If you generally eat a healthy diet but went out to celebrate last night, your triglyceride levels will be high, but your cholesterol may be low, for example.

How Fasting Can Affect Your Cholesterol Levels

Research shows how fasting can help reduce your levels of cholesterol and how it may be able to decrease your risks of coronary heart disease. One of these studies looked at whether alternate day fasting was able to reduce the risks of coronary heart disease. In this study, sixteen obese adults, four men, and 12 women participated in a ten-week study. Following eight weeks of treatment, the LDL in the patients was reduced by 25 percent while their triglyceride levels went down by 32 percent. In addition to these numbers, the fat mass, waist size, and body weight of the participants were reduced.

In another 12-week study, researchers looked at how exercise and diet affected HDL and LDL levels in obese adults. Most people who are obese will have a lipid profile that is high in LDL and HDL particles. There were 60 subjects, and they were randomly put into four groups. These four groups included those who did alternate day fasting, those who did calorie restriction, those who exercised and did moderate intensity training three times a week, and those in the control group.

Out of this study, researchers found that both diet and exercise had a similar effect on weight loss in the participants, but this affected HDL and LDL in different ways. Those on the alternate day fast and the calorie restriction group had a five percent reduction in weight loss and an increase in LDL, but there were no changes in HDL. In comparison, those who were in the exercise group lost five percent of body weight and saw improvements in their HDL, but no changes in LDL. What this shows is that it may be best to do a combination of diet and exercise so you can improve both types of cholesterol together.

What Are Some Ways to Lower Your Cholesterol?

•Avoid foods that are high in empty calories: Always pick out foods that are high in healthy nutrients and low in empty calories if you want to lose weight and pick foods that will keep you full so that you can lose weight as well as lower your cholesterol levels.

•Lose weight and add in more exercise: As some of the studies above show, exercise and diet combined can be the best way to help lower your bad cholesterol and increase the good cholesterol.

•Eat more protein and fiber: Protein and fiber can do wonders for keeping you full on fewer calories. Plus, a lot of the sources of these nutrients are low in bad fats that can increase your cholesterol levels.

•Avoid overeating and keep your portions small: Intermittent fasting can help with both. Even if you slightly overeat after your fast, the amount is not going to overcompensate for the calories that you missed. And since your eating window is usually smaller, it will be easier for you to keep your portions under control.

•Grilling, boiling, or baking your meals: Deep fat frying and other options than the three listed above can add lots of extra bad fats to your diet, which will increase your cholesterol levels. Try to use healthy cooking methods.

•Do an intermittent fast: Many people who go on an intermittent fast find that it is easier to control their calories and lose weight, which can be important to lower your cholesterol levels. It works the same in many studies as calorie restriction, but for most people, the intermittent fast is easier to maintain.

Chapter 9: Intermittent Fasting and Your Heart Health

So far, we have spent some time talking about the amazing benefits that can come with intermittent fasting. We have even talked about some of the ways that fasting can help improve the health of your heart, such as by lowering your cholesterol levels and reducing inflammation. Just by increasing your insulin sensitivity, intermittent fasting can help reduce your risk of heart disease by 93 percent.

When it comes to looking just at the heart and how healthy it is, many experts look at a variety of factors, including inflammatory markers, blood pressure, triglycerides, and cholesterol levels. And it just happens that intermittent fasting can help reduce all these risk factors. Let's look at how intermittent fasting can really help improve your heart health so that you can live a long and happy life.

How Does Intermittent Fasting Help with Circulation and Healthy Hearts?

Intermittent fasting can be very effective at reducing your risk of circulatory and heart disease. Cardiovascular diseases are one of the leading causes of death in the world, with one in six deaths in the United States attributed to heart disease and one in 19 deaths due to a stroke. Many people wrongly assume that heart disease only occurs in men, but women can be just as much, if not more, at risk of this disease.

There are a variety of risk factors that can lead to cardiovascular disease. Some of these include:

•Being overweight. This is particularly concerning if your waistline is larger and you carry more weight around your middle.

•Lack of exercise.

•Poor diet.

•Diabetes.

•Insulin resistance and a high level of glucose in the blood.

•High blood pressure.

•Smoking has been shown to cause several issues with your heart health. The chemicals that are found in cigarettes can easily cause the blood vessels to narrow, forcing the heart to pump blood harder than before.

Fasting can help with some of these risk factors. For example, it can help you to lose weight so that your weight and your waistline are no longer a big issue. It can help lower your blood pressure, reduce the risk that you have for diabetes, and can reduce insulin resistance. Fasting can even help you get on a healthier diet because your cravings for processed and junk foods will be reduced. If you add in a healthy lifestyle to this as well, you may be able to stop smoking and add in more exercise to help with those risk factors as well.

A Look at How Cardiovascular Disease Can Develop

Cardiovascular disease is a pretty general term that is used to discuss all of the diseases that can occur to your circulation and your heart. It can include coronary heart disease, like a heart attack or angina, heart failure, and even stroke. These diseases are all going to be caused when fatty deposits are allowed to build up in the arteries, a process that is known as atherosclerosis.

The exact cause of this is not always certain. Many people originally thought that it was obvious that having higher levels of fat in the blood would be the culprit of this issue. However, scientific research has shown that this is too easy, and it may not always be the case. The exact kinds of fats that you consume will be the important part. In addition, the amount of inflammation that is found in the arteries may be a factor as well. Carrying an excess amount of fat around the internal organs and having issues with resistance to insulin can also increase your risk of developing this condition.

What is known is that once fats build up in the arteries, they become narrower and stiffer. The result of this is an increase in your blood pressure because it takes more pressure to get the blood through your narrowed arteries. If this narrowing occurs too much, then there can be problems like angina, pain when walking, and even heart attacks. The heart is working hard to pump blood throughout the body, but if the arteries get completely blocked, then the organs, including the heart, won't be able to get the blood that they need to function.

This kind of health concern is going to occur over time, with an unhealthy lifestyle and diet. Many people may not realize the extent of their issues and will wait until it is too late to do something that will make it better. It is much better to work on a healthier lifestyle and diet as early as possible to ensure that you don't have to deal with any of the many cardiovascular diseases that can harm your body.

Is Intermittent Fasting Able to Reduce My Risk of Developing Cardiovascular Disease?

The good news is that many studies have found that intermittent fasting can improve the risk factors for cardiovascular disease. This means that when you are on a fast, you can reduce your risks of developing one of these diseases. Some risk factors, such as insulin resistance, cholesterol, blood pressure, and weight (particularly fat that is around your waist), can all be improved with intermittent fasting.

Individuals who went on a 24-hour fast just once a month were less likely to be diagnosed with coronary artery disease. This is based on a study of 448 people in Utah and those who fasted that was also suffering from type 2 diabetes. Imagine the changes that could happen if these individuals chose to fast for more than one day a month, such as doing the 5:2 diet or an alternate day fasting schedule. Their risk of developing cardiovascular disease may be even lower.

In addition, there were studies done on obese and overweight women who were asked to fast every other day for eight weeks. These participants were allowed to have about 500 calories a day on their fasting day. After the eight weeks were over, these women had lost weight and reduced their waist size, decreased their LDL and cholesterol, lowered their blood pressure, and more.

In a further study, it was found that these same kinds of improvements to cardiovascular health were also seen in people whether they ate on the traditional diet most Americans follow or a low-fat diet on their non-fasting days. Moreover, other studies that look at alternate day fasting have confirmed these benefits to the health of your heart.

Another research study showed that overweight women who did a semi-fast for two days a week, which meant they could eat up to 600 calories on their fasting days, had a reduction in insulin resistance, blood pressure, triglycerides, total and LDL cholesterol   , inflammation, and leptin. This shows that whether the women went on an alternate day fast or the 5:2 diet, they saw results that could improve the health of their heart.

Studies have also been done on daily fasting during Ramadan. These studies show that there was an improvement in cardiovascular risks with this type of fasting as well. Often, this form of fasting is not going to be used for the health benefits, though, and is done to follow a religion. Some studies may not encourage this form of fasting to keep you healthy for the long term.

To get some of the good benefits that come from intermittent fasting, you must take the time to eat a diet that is healthy and wholesome. If you go on one of these fasting choices and then spend your time eating a lot of junk and processed foods, it isn't going to help your risk of developing cardiovascular disease, and you will be in just as much trouble as before.

The exact way that intermittent fasting can cause beneficial changes to your cardiovascular risk is still unknown. However, it seems like some of the key factors include helping the individual to lose weight, improve their insulin resistance, and inflammation. The reduction in waist size can be a good indicator that you are heading in the right direction when it comes to reducing your risk of cardiovascular disease. If you have a large risk for cardiovascular disease or you have some of the risk factors discussed above, then it may be time to consider going on a 5:2 diet or an alternate day fast to help you get some results to cut down on your cardiovascular risk.

Chapter 10: Intermittent Fasting and Cancer

One benefit that you can get from intermittent fasting that may be surprising is that it can help protect you from, and fight against, cancer. Studies indicate that fasting can help reduce some of the side effects that come from chemotherapy, improve immunity, slow down the growth of cancerous tumors, and increase survival rates. This benefit still needs more research, but so far, it looks like intermittent fasting can be beneficial and safe for most cancer patients if it is done under the supervision of your doctor or medical professional.

How Can Intermittent Fasting Help Me Fight Cancer?

Fasting can help you fight cancer because it activates the immune system of the body. The immune system is designed to help find and then eliminate anything foreign that is present and could harm your health. However, it is not as effective at finding and then eliminating abnormal cells in the body, such as cancer cells. Intermittent fasting may be just what your immunity needs to become more effective at getting rid of these abnormal cells.

Research that was conducted at the University of Southern California showed that mice who fasted when they received chemotherapy ended up responding more favorably to treatment compared to mice who just went through chemo on its own. The mice that were on a fast produced more of the immune system cells, specifically the T cells and B cells, that were able to target and destroy both tumor cells and breast cancer cells. In addition, fasting can be helpful in making the drugs for chemotherapy more effective and could slow down the spread of cancer to other areas.

Researchers also found that going through many rounds of fasting, or at least more than one, could be enough to slow down the growth of human neuroblastoma, glioma, melanoma, and breast cancer. In some cases, it appears that fasting may be as effective as chemotherapy in treating some types of cancer in some patients.

One study on this had mice who were dealing with human ovarian cancer. The ones who had this and went on a fast ended up living longer than those who didn't fast. In fact, up to 20 percent of the mice who had a deadly form of children's neuroendocrine cancer was cured after doing several rounds of fasting combined with chemotherapy. Another 40 percent of mice showed the lesser spread of same cancer when they combined the two treatments together. In that same study, all the mice who only underwent chemotherapy died.

While studies are limited on how intermittent fasting can affect humans, one study has taken the time to look at the effectiveness, as well as the safety, of fasting while on chemotherapy. For this study, 20 patients with cancer were divided into three groups. One group fasted for 24 hours, one for 48, and the last for 72 hours before chemotherapy. The results of this showed that fasting helped to reduce insulin-like growth factor 1, which is a growth factor that has been linked to certain cancers. Even when the patients went back to their regular diet, the effect from the fast continued for 24 hours after the chemotherapy session ended.

Another neat thing to consider is that individuals who have Laron syndrome, which is a disorder that inhibits IGF-1 also have lower risks of developing diabetes and cancer compared to the general population. This is a similar thing that can happen when patients undergo a fast before chemotherapy. This fasting also helped limit DNA damage and less toxicity in healthy tissues after the chemotherapy treatment was done. The longer fasts seemed to be more effective.

In addition to all the great benefits and the effectiveness of fasting along with chemotherapy, patients who went on the fast found that they didn't undergo severe side effects. At worst, they suffered from dizziness, headaches, and fatigue, which could also happen from the chemotherapy treatment. They had no signs of malnutrition.

Can Fasting Help with Breast Cancer?

Breast cancer patients may be able to benefit from fasting as well. There is evidence that doing a fast or dealing with calorie restriction can help starve out the cancer cells and makes them respond better to chemotherapy. In addition, fasting could boost the immunity of the individual so it can fight off tumor growth and prevent cancer from spreading through the body.

In one study, researchers put mice who had breast cancer on a diet that mimicked a fast, one that was low in sugar, protein, and calories. The mice on this fast had their calories cut in half on the first day, and then the next three days their calories were cut by 9.7 percent. After four days of this diet, the mice were allowed to eat in a normal way for ten days before going on the fast again. This repeated a few times.

Mice who went on this fasting diet had reductions in the cell growth of their breast cancer, even though they didn't go on chemotherapy in that time. Their cancer cells became more sensitive to chemotherapy drugs as well, and their bodies were more effective at finding, targeting, and then destroying tumor growth. After three rounds of this fasting cycle, along with the doxorubicin chemotherapy drugs, the white blood cells of the mice increased by 33 percent. This is an important thing to note since these white blood cells are needed to help the body fight cancer.

But what about the results in humans? One study that was done through the University of California looked at whether daily fasts could help reduce the risks and recurrence of breast cancer. The study took self-reported data from 2,413 women who had early-stage breast cancer between 1995 and 2007. The participants ranged in ages between 27 to 70, and they would fast for an average of 12.5 hours a night.

The women in this study who fasted for 13 hours or less each night ended up having a higher risk of breast cancer recurrence compared to the women who fasted over 13 hours each night. For every increase of two hours in the duration of a nightly fast, there was lower blood sugar levels and a longer duration of nighttime sleep. The report also noted how fasting could help protect against heart disease and type 2 diabetes.

Can Fasting Help Reduce the Side Effects of Chemotherapy?

In addition to helping you fight cancer, fasting can help you get through the side effects of chemotherapy easier. In one study that was done, cancer patients who fasted for a maximum of five days and then had a normal diet before treatment reported that they had fewer side effects compared to those who didn't fast before treatment. They also reported less gastrointestinal issues, less weakness and fatigue, reduced cramps and numbness, fewer headaches, and no vomiting. Moreover, the fasting didn't make them lose an unsafe amount of weight or interfere at all with their treatment.

However, there are a few concerns that have come with intermittent fasting for a cancer patient. The biggest one is that it may cause additional weight loss in a patient who is already at risk for weight loss. While weight loss is good for someone who is obese or overweight, in a cancer patient, it is not a good thing.

Some patients may also have issues with dizziness, headache, weakness, and fatigue because of fasting. And since the patient is already dealing with being in a weaker state due to their treatments, this may make things worse. Therefore, patients who are considering using a fast during their cancer treatment should discuss this option with a doctor before they start. If the doctor and the patient think this is a good option, then the patient must make sure that they start with a shorter fast and slowly extend the duration to see whether the effectiveness is increased.

If a cancer patient is going to go on a longer fast, one that is more than a day or two, then this fast needs to be monitored by a doctor. This will ensure that the patient is getting the nutrition that they need during the fast and that this fast won't mess with their treatment at all. When the patient is not on a fast, they should make sure they eat a well-balanced diet that has a ton of nutrition and whole foods, as well as lower the consumption of refined carbs and eat more protein.

More research needs to be done to help determine whether fasting can be an effective way to help treat cancer and to make sure that the side effects of chemotherapy and other cancer treatments are kept to a minimum. However, with the animal studies and a few reviews that have been done so far, fasting may be the answer that many cancer patients have been waiting for.

Chapter 11: Intermittent Fasting and Epilepsy

Fasting has been used for centuries to help naturally treat the body for many conditions. And now, it may be possible to use intermittent fasting, especially when it is combined with the ketogenic diet, as an effective way to help fight epilepsy. While studies are still out on whether intermittent fasting can help epilepsy effectively on its own, it is very effective when it works with the ketogenic diet.

Early evidence has shown that abstaining from carbs and going on a water fast could help reduce the frequency of epileptic seizures for more than half the patients who were given the fasting based therapy, according to research that has been done at Johns Hopkins University. This is a powerful look at the fact that intermittent fasting may be able to help treat epilepsy, especially for children who rely on medication to provide them some relief from epilepsy.

What Is Epilepsy?

Epilepsy is a chronic disorder where unprovoked and recurrent seizures are normal. A person who suffers epilepsy is classified as one who has two unprovoked seizures that weren't caused by some reversible or known medical condition. For example, if someone had a seizure because their blood sugars got low or they were having withdrawals from alcohol, then they would not be considered epileptic.

The seizures that occur in epilepsy can be related to family tendency and brain injury in some cases, but often the cause is not known. Many people who suffer from this disorder may have more than one type of seizure and other neurological problems.

Although the symptoms of these seizures can affect any part of the body, the events that cause the seizures, including the electrical events, are going to occur in the brain. The location of that event, how far it spreads, and how much of your brain is going to be affected can all have effects on the individual. Sometimes the seizure is smaller and won't cause many issues, but over time, these instances often get worse, and the side effects will grow.

The Ketogenic Diet and Fat Burning

The ketogenic diet is very different from the traditional diet plan that most Americans follow. While many Americans follow a diet that is all about eating lots of carbs and plenty of processed foods, the ketogenic diet relies more on eating lots of healthy fats and keeping the carb content down as much as possible.

As the body switches off from eating carbs and having a constant source of easy glucose to use as fuel, it instead starts to rely on fat as its main source of energy. The body will then start to enter ketosis. The ketones that are produced from that is going to trigger some small biochemical changes in the brain, changes that can be very beneficial to patients who have epilepsy. Trials, as well as observations, show how the ketogenic diet can help at least half of the epilepsy patients who decide to try it and 20 percent of patients are going to see some huge improvements.

While more studies need to be done to see if the ketogenic diet can make changes in the brain that can benefit those with epilepsy, early research shows that the process that goes on during the ketogenic diet can actually help those with this disorder. It is a simple change to make and can definitely help one to avoid seizures.

Fasting May Be a Good Stand-Alone Therapy for Epilepsy

In another study that was done at Johns Hopkins University, there was further evidence of the benefits of using the ketogenic diet along with periodic fasting. This study also showed that these two approaches can complement each other and that using them together can provide the best results. A pediatric neurologist from Johns Hopkins University, Adam Hartman, explains that the current evidence suggests that fasting is not just enhancing the effects of the ketogenic diet in epileptic patients, but it could also be enough to change up the metabolism of children with epilepsy and could be used as a stand-alone therapy for some patients.

In the current study, researchers tested children who went on just the ketogenic diet on its own, and they achieved only moderate results. The children then went on a fast along with the ketogenic diet, and at the end of this, four out of six children who were tested reported that they had fewer seizures.

This helps to prove that fasting may be a good stand-alone treatment for children who are suffering from epilepsy and drug-resistant. The latest study shows that even those who only saw a little bit of relief with the ketogenic diet were able to see some significant results when they started to introduce periodic fasting to the mix as well. Hartman and other researchers plan to focus studies in the future on determining how intermittent fasting can affect seizures and whether fasting would be an effective method to help control certain types of seizures.

Chapter 12: Intermittent Fasting and Improving Your Mind and Preventing Neurodegenerative Diseases

Anything that you do that is good for your body is bound to be good for the brain as well. Intermittent fasting has been shown to improve a variety of metabolic features that are super important when it comes to the health of your brain. This can include things like reducing inflammation, reducing issues with insulin resistance, reducing blood sugar levels, and reducing oxidative stress throughout the body.

There have been several animal studies that show how intermittent fasting can help increase how fast nerve cells can grow. The faster that these nerve cells can grow, the easier it is for the brain to stay sharp and focused no matter what you are working on. Moreover, intermittent fasting can increase the levels of BDNF, or brain-derived neurotrophic factor, in order to fight off various brain problems such as depression. It is no wonder that intermittent fasting is recommended for improving the brain.

There are so many great benefits that come from following an intermittent fast. Many people will see a reduction in some neurodegenerative diseases, an increase in their focus and concentration, and so much more. Let's take a closer look at how intermittent fasting can help protect your brain!

How Intermittent Fasting Helps to Improve the Way That Our Brains Function

One of the most common things that people want to improve on is their concentration and focus at work and in other parts of their life. Fatigue, brain fog, and an inability to keep themselves on task can be common symptoms that people in all industries face each day. Add in some issues like weight gain, high insulin levels, and high blood sugars and our ability to concentrate on the task at hand diminishes further.

Intermittent fasting may be the answer that you are looking for if you need to fight off brain fog and fatigue and you want to be able to concentrate and focus. One recent study showed that when overweight mice went on an intermittent fast, it helped them much better with learning and memory scores. There was also a big improvement in the structural function of their brains. It is a nice combination; a slimmer waistline and better brain function all rolled into one package!

What this means is that by going on an intermittent fast, even by fasting a few days a week, you are greatly improving the overall functioning of your brain. You are clearing out the brain so that it can remember more so that it can focus, and so that concentration is easier than ever before.

Intermittent Fasting and Alzheimer's Disease

Alzheimer's disease is one of the most common neurodegenerative diseases in the whole world. There is no cure available for this disease right now, so the best thing to do is learn how to prevent it in the first place. In one study that was done on rats, it was shown that intermittent fasting might be able to delay Alzheimer's in those who don't have it and reduce the severity in those who already suffer from the disease.

In a series of reports that were done, a lifestyle intervention that had short-term fasts done every day was able to help improve the symptoms of Alzheimer's in nine out of ten patients. In addition, several animal studies suggest that fasting may be able to help with some other neurodegenerative disease, such as Huntington's and Parkinson's disease.

Helps Fight off Depression

Depression and other low mood disorders are quickly rising throughout the world. In fact, this has become such a big issue that the World Health Organization predicts that by 2030, depression is going to be the leading cause of disease burden throughout the whole world. More people than ever are fighting off depression and other mood disorders, and this could be a major problem.

One root cause of depression and low mood could be chronically high insulin and blood sugar levels. The hormones that are affected by these two things, which can also lead to a rise in type 2 diabetes, are also going to affect the hormones that are in control of our moods. With the average sugar consumption at 160 pounds per year per person, it is no wonder that this is a big issue that many people are facing right now.

The best thing to do is work on reducing your high blood sugar and insulin levels. We have already shown how intermittent fasting can help make this happen. By going on a fast and changing up some of the hormones in the body during the process, while also reducing the amount of sugar and refined carbs we take in, not only are we reducing our risk of type 2 diabetes, but we are also working on helping to improve our mood and fight off depression.

Fasting May Be Able to Protect the Brain Against Disease

In addition to all the benefits that we have discussed in this guidebook, fasting may have the power to help protect your brain against various degenerative illnesses. Researchers from the National Institute of Ageing have found evidence that states how periodic fasting or fasting for just one or two days each week, may protect your brain from the effects of Parkinson's, Alzheimer's and other ailments.

When you reduce the number of calories that you take in, it may help your brain. However, doing regular calorie restriction may not be enough to make this happen. It is much better to go on an intermittent fast, or periodically cut out meals in your week, rather than just restricting your calories. Then implement some days where you can eat as much as you want. What this means is that timing is a very crucial element when it comes to how well you can protect your brain.

Cutting daily food intake to about 500 calories for that day, which is going to be a small meal, for two days out of the week, can have some beneficial effects on your brain and how strong it can stay. It is as simple as adding one or two fasting days to your week, and then eating as normally as possible the rest of the week so that you can protect against some neurodegenerative diseases in the body.

Many scientists have known for a long time that eating a diet that is lower in calories can help you lead a longer life. Mice and rats that were raised on restricted amounts of food were able to increase their lifespan 40 percent or more compared to those who didn't restrict their calories. And this same effect has been seen in humans.

But now research is taking this idea a little bit further. It is now argued that by having an occasional fast and not eating as much for one or two days during the week is not going to cause early death or even ill health. However, it could help delay the onset of conditions that could affect the brain, even for conditions like stroke, Parkinson's and Alzheimer's.

The reason that this may work is that the growth of neurons in the brain may be most affected when you reduce the amount of energy that you take in. The amounts of the messaging chemicals between two cells will be boosted when you sharply reduce the number of calories that you consume. These chemical messengers are going to play an important role in boosting the growth of neurons in the brain, something that would be able to counteract how impactful Parkinson's and Alzheimer's are.

The link between boosting cell growth in the brain and reductions in the amount of energy you take in may seem unlikely, but there are some evolutionary reasons for believing in this. In the past, when resources were scarce, our ancestors would need to scrounge around and find food. Those who had brains that could respond well to this, the ones who could remember where promising sources of food were or how to avoid predators, would be the ones who got to the food and survived. This is how this link was developed.

Currently, more studies need to be done on the effect, and researchers, including those at Johns Hopkins University, are getting ready to take it further. They are preparing to study how fasting can impact the brain through MRI scans and other techniques. If the results come back the way that most studies have shown so far, it is possible that the missing link to protecting your brain and your mental health is intermittent fasting.

Chapter 13: Are There Any Negative Side Effects of Going on an Intermittent Fast?

Below are some of the negative side effects of going on an intermittent fast:

•Feeling full after you break your fast and eat.

Our bodies generally follow an unhealthy eating plan. We are used to eating at least three big meals a day and then lots of snacks any time that we feel a bit hungry, when we get near a mealtime, or just have a craving. Because we are used to eating that often, the body learns to expect food at certain times. The ghrelin hormone is responsible for making us feel hungry, and it is set up to peak during the main meal times. It is often regulated by the food that we take in.

•Becoming really obsessed with your eating and fasting windows.

When we decide to go on a fast, the ghrelin levels are still going to peak at the same times that they did before. Even though we aren't eating, and we are going to be just fine moving our meal times around, these levels will peak at breakfast, lunch, and dinner, and we will feel very hungry when they do. Often, days three to five of the fast are going to be the hardest. If you can stick with this for a week or so and adjust your body and the ghrelin levels to eating at different times, the hunger will naturally go away.

•Lots of cravings and hunger.

One option that you can try out when you want to fight off those hunger pains and make sure that you don't give in during your fasting window is to make sure that you take in a lot of water during that time. Water can help fill up the stomach and make you feel more alert. And for some people, the action of just putting something in their mouth to eat, or in this case drink, when they are hungry, can be enough to make the hunger pains go away.

If you need something that is a bit different than water to enjoy during your fasting time to get rid of hunger, you can consider black coffee or drinking some tea. This can help to curb your hunger. Keep yourself busy as well to help you not think about the hunger as much. You can work out, clean the house, or just find something that you enjoy doing.

When it is time to get back to your eating window, you need to make some plans. You must make sure that this time is full of healthy nutrients, and that you are taking in enough calories so that you can fill up. This will easily make a difference in how much hunger you feel during your fasting period.

•Heartburn

•Headaches

As your body gets used to going on an intermittent fast, there are times when the body will experience a dull headache, one that isn't constant but comes and goes. There are different reasons that this may happen, including dehydration if you don't make sure you are drinking enough fluids during your fasting window. It is a good idea to monitor your fluids and always keep a water bottle nearby. When you aren't eating, it is easy to forget that you need to drink, and dehydration and the headaches that accompany it can sneak up on you.

Not only can dehydration cause headaches, but you could experience headaches because of a decrease in your blood sugar levels. Some people experience more stress hormones released in the brain when they decide to fast as well. The good news is that these go away quickly. Just make sure that you drink plenty of water during the day, keep some painkillers around, and take it slowly for the first few days.

•Brain fog in the beginning.

•Can negatively affect the hormones of women.

Some women find that they are going to react negatively to the changes in the amount they eat. For some women, this is not a big issue, and they can change the way that they eat without many issues to start with. However, for some women, changing up the way they eat and any sign that they are going into starvation mode can cause issues with their hormones and can slow down the metabolism.

We will talk about this topic more in a future chapter. Women are often very sensitive to changes in the way that they eat. To preserve the reproductive system, women are going to respond differently to these fasts compared to men, and they need to be careful about how they go on one of these fasts to start with.

•Fatigue

During the first few days, and up to a week, that you are on an intermittent fast, you may feel overly tired. Many people worry that they are doing the fast the wrong way or that it isn't for them because they are so tired when they first get started. The important thing here is just to keep going with the fast and realize that feeling tired in the beginning is completely normal.

When you think about everything that happens when you are on a fast, it shouldn't surprise you as much that you feel so tired at first. With your traditional diet, your body relies much on processed carbs and sugars that are turned into glucose in the body. Glucose is a very easy source of energy, one that the body will actively search for. However, our bodies don't effectively burn through the glucose that we eat, and much of it gets stored as body fat, even as we crave more of it.

With intermittent fasting, we take away that easy source of energy for longer periods of time. The body must learn how to find good sources of energy that aren't glucose to keep us up and running, and this can be hard. For some who had poor eating habits before the fast, it can be hard for the body to know what to go after for fuel.

While the body searches around for the energy that it needs, it is going to be tired. You are going to feel worn down and like you just want to sleep all day long. But it will only take the body a few days before it will start to use the stored glycogen or the stored body fat as fuel, and you will get the energy back. Until that time, take it easy, avoid being around anything that will stress you out or cause you to be irritable (high irritability and low tolerance for stress are common while fasting), and you will be just fine.

For the most part, these negative side effects are just going to be temporary. As the body adjusts to this new form of eating, you will get used to them and won't have to deal with them as much. Just stick it out, and after a week or so on a fasting regimen, you are going to notice a big difference with most side effects gone.

Chapter 14: Men vs. Women – Why Women Should Fast Differently Than Men

Following an intermittent fast can be a great way to help you increase your metabolism, reduce your calories, and lose weight while improving your health all at once. There are many ways that you can go on an intermittent fast, and with all those methods, it's easy for everyone to get on this fast and make it work for their lifestyle. However, women often have to follow some special rules when they go on an intermittent fast to avoid sensitivities to these eating changes that can mess with their hormones and cause problems.

The way that men and women fast will be different, and many times, women will need to take caution and be careful when they decide to fast.

Many women have been worried about going on an intermittent fast because they are worried about issues with metabolic disruptions, menstrual periods, and more from this kind of fasting. Thus, women are going to respond differently to men with these fasts.

This doesn't mean that women aren't able to see results though. It just means that you need to be careful about the way that you fast, and take it slowly, to get the best results. This chapter is going to look at some of the basics that you can follow as a woman on an intermittent fast to get the best results.

As a woman, when you decide to go on an intermittent fast, you must be careful about the method you choose, how much you fast, and the number of calories and nutrition that you take in each day. Women are often sensitive to changes in their diet and even when they get enough nutrition and calories while fasting, the longer periods of not eating may adversely affect them.

Women can still go on an intermittent fast and see some great results, but they do need to take some extra precautions to make sure they are doing it in a manner that is safe and effective for them. For some women, these precautions aren't necessary, and they will be able to go on a fast and not have any negative effects. For other women, this chapter will help them to make sure that they listen to their bodies and stay safe while they are on their fast.

What Happens to the Hormones of Women During Fasting?

Intermittent fasting may not seem like a big deal to most people. They may think that getting into it and experimenting a bit isn't going to make that big of a difference. But for some women, these small decisions can have a huge impact. The hormones in women that are responsible for regulating key functions in women, including ovulation and reproduction, can be sensitive regarding the energy that you take in.

In both genders, the hypothalamic-pituitary-gonadal axis, which is the cooperative functioning of three endocrine glands, can act like an air traffic controller. First, your hypothalamus is going to release a hormone that is known as GnRH. This is then going to tell your pituitary gland to release the LH hormone and the FHS hormone.

These two hormones are going to act on the gonads of the individual, which would be either the ovaries or the testes. In women, this means that these hormones are going to trigger the production of progesterone and estrogen, both of which are needed to help release a mature egg and to help support a pregnancy. For men, these hormones are going to trigger the production of testosterone and sperm production.

This reaction is supposed to happen at a specific time to help the cycle in women stay as regular as possible. To make this happen, the pulses of GnRH must be timed so that everything goes at the right time. However, the problem comes in because these pulses are very sensitive to factors in the environment. And if you don't pay attention to your body and what is going on, these things can sometimes be thrown off through fasting. Even a short-term fast can end up causing many issues for women.

Why Does Fasting Seem to Affect Women More Than Men?

Many studies are unsure about why intermittent fasting affects women more than men. One thought is that it has to do with the levels of kisspeptin in women versus men. This is a molecule neurons use to communicate with each other. This hormone is going to stimulate the production of GnRH in both sexes, and it will have a very high sensitivity to insulin, leptin, and ghrelin hormones that are responsible for regulating hunger and satiety.

One interesting thing is that females produce higher levels of this hormone compared to men. And the more of this hormone in the body, the higher the sensitivity to any changes in energy balance. This may be a good clue as to why many women have trouble going into one of these fasts.

For many women who go on a fast, the best solution that you can try out is to limit the amount of time that you go on a fast to start with.

Doing options like either the 5:2 diet or the 16/8 diet are often best, but women should avoid options like the warrior diet.

Are There Any Times When I Should Stop Doing an Intermittent Fast?

Remember that many women are going to be sensitive to changes in eating. While most women can avoid issues simply by slowly entering their intermittent fast, other women may find that intermittent fasting is not for them and they need to try something else. When certain symptoms begin, it is the body's way of telling you that things need to change. Many of these symptoms can lead to serious conditions and health concerns in the future. Some of the signs that intermittent fasting is causing worse than good and that it is time to stop your fasting include:

- You are always cold and can't warm yourself up.

- You notice that your digestive system has slowed down.

- You have no interest in a romantic life, especially if you had a good romance life before the fast.

- Your heart is going to feel like it is making strange beats. Watch out for any rapid beats at random times.

- You have lots of mood swings, and they seem like they are all over the place.

- You notice that when any stress comes up in your life, your tolerance is low, and you just can't seem to handle it at all.

- If you end up getting injured during your time trying out a fast, and you have a lot of trouble healing. In addition, you catch a bug and have trouble fighting it off, no matter what is going around.

- When you finish up with a workout while fasting and are struggling to recover from it. If you used to work out and you start to have trouble with recovering once you start fasting, that is something to watch out for as well.

•You notice that your skin is very dry when you fast and nothing seems to help.

•You see that your hair is falling out.

•It is hard for you to fall asleep and even when you do fall asleep, it is hard for you to stay asleep at night.

•You notice that your menstrual cycle is changing. It may be irregular for more than one month, or you notice that you miss your cycle for a few months in a row (and you are not pregnant).

If you start to notice that a few of these conditions are affecting you, then it may be time to make some changes to your fasting schedule. If you are on an alternate day fast, then maybe move back to the eat stop eat method or 16/8 method to help you lose weight. These are easier on the system and won't affect your hormone levels at all. If you were already on one of those, then it may be time to stop intermittent fasting altogether.

Chapter 15: What Should I Expect When I Get Started with Fasting?

Once you have gotten started with fasting, you may be nervous about what to expect. Most of us have rarely ever missed a meal unless we were sick, and we have spent most of our lives being told that fasting is very bad for our health. Even with knowing all the great health benefits that have been discussed in this guidebook, it can still be a little hard to understand what is going to happen when you start your fast.

For the first few fasts that you undertake, the situation may be difficult. If you can get through the first two or three, then things get easier, but be ready for a rough couple of days as you start to adjust. The hunger that bothers you, in the beginning, will start to dissipate a bit and can be quelled with the help of a drink of water. You may also deal with a few other issues, such as headaches and heartburn like we talked about before, but these often disappear after a few fasts.

Some people are going to experience more issues with their fast compared to others. No one is quite sure why some people have bigger problems, but it may have to do with the diet that you had before you began fasting. One cause of fasting being more difficult for some compared to others is a phenomenon that is known as metabolic inflexibility. This is when the body has become so used to that constant supply of carbs and sugar from food that it is out of practice, turning to our fat stores for energy, and the side effects can hit you hard. However, the body is very adaptive, and after just a few fasts, it will learn how to access those fat stores to keep you energized, and the side effects are going to fade.

There are a few different problems that a beginner faster may experience. Some of these include:

> •Intense hunger: These hunger pains will come and go through the day. These pains are like waves, rather than something that just builds up, so you just need to find ways to distract yourself to make it easier.

> •Headaches: These are common when you first start. Take some painkillers to help and drink plenty of fluids.

> •Lightheadedness: Some people report feeling a bit lightheaded and spaced out when they go on a fast. When you get to your eating window, eat something a little bit salty.

> •Feeling tired: This is going to happen because the body hasn't had time to learn how to access the stores of fat that you have as fuel. A salty drink can help with this.

> •Lots of irritability: This can be a big problem when you are near the end of your fast. Planning out the meals that you are going to eat ahead of time can really help. Be aware that your temper may be short, learn how to stay calm or stay away from other people.

•Insomnia: Some people have trouble falling asleep when they go on their first few fasts.

The good news is that most of these are going to fade away within a week or less. Having a good meal plan when you first get started on your intermittent fast and sticking with it, can make a big difference in how well you feel and how successful the fast is. When meal planning, add in lots of nutrients and consider putting one of your bigger meals as the first one to help the body get enough food after going on the fast.

There are also a few things that you can do to reduce the side effects of an intermittent fast and help you be better prepared for this kind of eating plan. First, take it easy for the first few weeks. If you have a big project that is going to occur at work or another stressful situation at hand, then hold off getting started with intermittent fasting.

These situations are going to make you crave food all the time and can already give you headaches and irritability. Adding the intermittent fast on top of that will just make things worse. Consider taking a few days off work if you can or just pick a time that is less stressful and demanding on you to help you get the best results!

Meal planning is another option that you can choose. After you get done with a fast, especially during the first few times, you are going to be really hungry. The body is not used to going such a long time without eating, and as soon as you let it have something, it will want to gobble down as much as it can get ahold of. If you don't have a plan in place, you are going to eat everything in the kitchen and take on way too many calories in the process.

With a good meal plan, you can avoid this issue. You can set up your meals ahead of time, especially for those eating periods right after your fast is ending. That way, when the fast is done, you can just grab the prepared meal and enjoy it, knowing that the meal has all the good nutrients that your body needs and will fill you up.

One thing to remember about meal planning with intermittent fasting is to consider making the first meal after a fast a little bit bigger. Many of us save supper as our biggest meal, but when you are done with a fast, the body is hungry and has been going for a long time without anything to eat. You can certainly provide yourself with a tiny meal after the fast, but you will end up hungry and dissatisfied. A better option is to add a bit more to that first meal to help provide the body with nutrients and to make it feel better. This can make the fast more enjoyable and will ensure you don't go and raid the fridge simply because you are still hungry after your fast.

Chapter 16: Keeping the Fast: What Is Allowed When I Am Fasting?

Many people wonder what they are allowed to eat during their fasted state. They understand that they need to avoid drinks with calories and food and snacks during this time. However, what about some of the items that may not be considered as food, such as gum, breath mints, and even medications? These can provide a type of gray area when it comes to intermittent fasting.

The type of fast that you follow is going to determine what you can have and still maintain for the fast. For example, the regular alternate day fast would have you eat nothing on your fasting days, but the modified version allows you to have up to 500 calories during those fasting days.

On all forms, though, when you are fasting and not eating the one meal allowed, you are required to abstain from food and any drinks that have extra sugars and calories. Let's take a closer look at what is allowed when you are fasting and how to make sure you maintain your fasted state.

The Fasted State

With most forms of an intermittent fast, you will be required to separate your eating and fasting periods. During the eating periods, you are allowed to eat the amount of whole and nutritious foods that the body needs to stay healthy. The more that you can fill up on wholesome foods, the better you will feel when you get to your fasting window again. Focus on whole grains, lean protein, lots of fruits and vegetables, and some healthy dairy products if you can have them. Limit junk and processed food as much as possible.

When you are fasting, though, you need to maintain the fast. You should not eat anything during the fasting portion of this eating program. This allows the body to get into the fat burning state that it needs and can help you to cut down on calories. You can drink as much coffee, tea, and water as you would like to ensure that you stay hydrated.

When it comes to fasting, everything except the liquids that we mentioned before should be avoided. If special circumstances affect you, then you can take that into consideration and make some changes to your fast. But this is an exception and not the rule. For most people who go on an intermittent fast, it is best just to avoid eating anything and only consume the beverages that are listed above to ensure you don't enter dehydration.

If you can put something in your mouth, then it is often going to be considered as something that you should have while you are on your fast. This can include any food and snacks as well as breath mints, gum, and so on. Some fasting protocols may allow for you to consume these products and not consider it as breaking your fast. However, for the most part, it is best to abstain from anything except the non-caloric beverages. Exceptions can be made to things like medication. If you need to take a certain medication each day, you may want to consider following the 5:2 diet or modified alternate fast so that you can take some food in along with your medication to avoid making yourself sick in the process. Supplements and other similar products should be avoided as well until you can eat something with them.

The idea of bulletproof coffee has been introduced recently, and many people wonder if it should be counted as something that breaks the fast. It is coffee, which is one of the beverages allowed during your fast, but this kind of coffee adds in other ingredients that add to your calorie count.

In most instances, you would count it as something that breaks your fast because it does contain other food items and calories as well. You could easily introduce it with the first meal you consume during the day and get the same results. However, if your protocol says that it is not breaking the fast, then it is fine to follow that rule of thumb as well.

The 5:2 Diet and Modified Alternate Fasting

With the modified alternate day fast and the 5:2 diet, there are slightly different rules. These methods do allow you to eat a little bit on your fasting day, but you must keep this to a minimum. You are not allowed to graze on them, and you can't just eat whatever you want, or you will end up back to your original state.

On both versions of intermittent fasting, you can consume up to 500 calories each day. With the 5:2 diet, most people will choose to go with two meals during the day that are 250 calories each. With the modified alternate fasting diet, it is recommended that you eat just one meal, preferably towards the end of the fast or before going to bed, that totals 500 calories. Both can be effective, so you can choose the method that works for you.

When you do eat on both modified versions, you need to make sure that your meals are as nutritious as possible. You will quickly find that eating a bunch of junk is not going to fill you up and can make your fast even more miserable when cravings begin. Think about it.

Two donuts equal 500 calories; however, they are definitely not as filling and nutritious as some turkey or chicken, half a cup of fruit, half a cup of vegetables, and a glass of milk or another similar meal. Choose your meals wisely, and you won't feel as deprived when you are on the fast.

Outside of the 500 calories that you can consume on these modified versions, you need to stick with the same rules as the other fats. You are not allowed to eat anything during the fast. Supplements are often discouraged and should be saved for your eating window to avoid upsetting the stomach. Sodas and other sugary beverages should be avoided, but having water, tea, and coffee is just fine. If you have medications that you must take at certain times, then those are fine, but if you have some freedom in when to take them, wait until your eating window begins again.

Chapter 17: How Do I Track My Progress When I Fast?

When you go on an intermittent fast, you want to see results. But how do you know when you are actually seeing results? Just by looking in the mirror each day, it can be hard to see the results when they happen. Here are a few ways that you can track your progress so that any time you want to check up on yourself, or when you need some extra motivation, you can see how far you have come.

Take Progress Pictures

No one wants to take pictures of themselves when they are at the start of their weight loss journal. However, no matter how uncomfortable it may make you feel to take that picture when you are out of shape, knowing where you are when you get started with fasting, or with any kind of diet plan, can be essential. It is easy for many people just to rely on the scale and let it be the one in charge, but when you consider issues like bodyweight distribution, lean mass gains, and water weight, just looking at the number on the scale can make you miss out on many good changes that are occurring.

Taking the picture is very important. Yes, you do look in the mirror each day already, but since you already do this at least one time a day, the changes that occur are going to be pretty much imperceptible. You need to take the pictures to ensure that you are actually able to see the changes.

Pictures are nice because they give you some separation from the mirror to actually see what is going on. They can allow you to see where you started from and then compare that to where you are now. You can even put the pictures side by side and see if this proves that there are some big changes that have been occurring over time.

When you are getting started on an intermittent fast, make sure that you take pictures of your front, the sides, and the back. Then every few weeks to every month, take these same pictures again. Do not suck in your stomach or push it out; simply stay relaxed and keep the conditions between one picture set to another as similar as you can. This makes it easier to get accurate results and see what is going on. If possible, make sure that you wear the same outfit, take the pictures near the same time of day as each other, and try to stick with the same lighting and angles.

After you have been on your intermittent fast for a few months, take out these pictures and compare them side by side. While you may have been looking into the mirror and not noticing any differences, these pictures should tell a different story. If you followed the intermittent fast the right way and stuck with a healthy diet, you will be able to tell the difference from one picture set to the next, and the difference between the first set of pictures and where you are right now.

Retest the Benchmarks That You Make

This one is often used when it comes to weight lifting, but you can do it with other options as well. Let's look at weightlifting first. When you first get started, take some time to test your strength benchmarks. Check and see how much you can pull and press. What are your squat numbers? This gives you a good idea of your baseline for strength, and then you can figure out which numbers are the most achievable for you to work on. If you ever feel discouraged or like you are not progressing, go back to those benchmark numbers and see how easy they are and how much you can surpass them. You may be surprised at how much stronger you have gotten.

You can do this with any kind of workout. If you were starting to do walking as an exercise, see how fast you can do a mile and then test yourself to see if you could pick up the speed. If you were just starting out and your limit for working out was two miles or 30 minutes of cardio, push it and see how far you can go the next time that you are discouraged.

Make sure that you write these numbers down. They can be great indicators of your current strength, and you can use them to check whether you are getting stronger or not. Many times, we think we are stuck because we aren't able to hit a particularly hard goal. But then we go back and test ourselves, and we find that things really did change; we just didn't notice.

Bring out the Tape Measure

You may be relying on the scale to let you know if you are progressing or not, but it is important to remember that not all the weight you lose is going to be fat. To see if you are actually starting to become leaner and have progressed, even when the scale doesn't seem to want to move, you should bring out a tape measure. Some areas that you can track include your shoulders, biceps, thighs, waist, hips, and chest.

Knowing the measurements around your body could do more than just help you have a physique that is proportionate. Where you store much of your fat can be a big warning sign of complications that are related to obesity. These include things like heart disease, stroke, and diabetes. You can use these measurements to help learn your waist to hip ratio and determine whether you are at a higher risk of these issues as well.

Since intermittent fasting is meant to help you not only lose weight but also lose body fat, the tape measure option is a great idea   .

Sometimes, the scale is not going to move in the direction that you want it to, and this can be frustrating. However, when you record your measurements on a regular basis, you will see changes in the body, even if the scale is not going the way that you want.

To help you keep track of your own personal measurements, get a journal and write down the date and the measurements for at least your arms, hips, and waist. You can measure any other part of the body that you would like as well to keep you on track. Just hold the tape measure against the skin and measure around, but don't pull it tight or do anything that might give you an inaccurate number.

You should check these measurements on a regular basis. Once a month is a great timeline because it gives you enough time to see some results. If you would like to measure more often or do it every few months, then this is fine as well. Just make sure that you pick out a time limit that is far enough apart, but not too far, so you can actually see your results.

How Much Energy Do You Have Now?

Another benefit that you can get when you go on an intermittent fast is more energy. Once you are done with the first few weeks of your fast, and you can get the body adjusted to this new eating schedule, you are going to see a ton of energy in your daily life. Measuring the amount of energy that you have as you progress on your intermittent fast can help you better track how well the fast is working.

The best way to monitor this is to take a few minutes to journal it. Start a week or so before you decide to go on a fast. Describe how much energy you had, what your mood was like for the day and a few other notes. Then, keep this process up as you start the intermittent fast. Over the next month or so, keep writing. When the time is up, or any time that you want, look back at the notes that you made and see what a difference there is in your mood, energy levels, and outlook on life.

Your Health Markers

Regular visits to the doctor can also help you determine whether you are making progress with your intermittent fast. You can get important tests done, such as a diabetes screening and cholesterol check and then compare the numbers. Many people find that they have more success when they get their doctor on board with them. Before you go on an intermittent fast, consider going in for a checkup with your doctor and getting some easy tests done to see where your numbers are.

After you have been on the fast for six months or so, go back to your doctor and get those numbers checked again. If you were doing a good job staying on your fast and eating healthy foods during your eating window, you are going to be pleasantly surprised by the results that you get when you go back to the doctor.

Measure Your Body Fat

Another way that you can check out whether the intermittent fast is working for you is to measure your body fat. Remember that one of the benefits of going on an intermittent fast is that you get the benefit of losing a lot of belly fat in addition to weight. When you take the time to measure your body fat, you can see just how effective the eating plan is.

Skinfold measurements are a great way to estimate the percentage of fat that is on your body based on the fat that is present underneath the skin. While you may not be happy with the number that you see when you first get started, it is still a good idea to do this measurement because it gives you a place to start when you are dieting.

Keep in mind that sometimes the results can be off by up to six percent. However, if you do the same method each time that you do this, then the percentage loss trend can make it easier to see your progress when it comes to the amount of fat that you lose.

Try on Some Old Clothing

If you are on an intermittent fast and you feel that you have plateaued, or you just want to see how far you have come, then taking out some of your old clothes and trying them on can help you get a good perspective on how far you have come. Sure, you may not have hit the goal that you set, but when you put on a pair of old jeans that used to be tight, and now you are swimming in them, it can certainly make you feel good! While it is a good idea to get rid of many of your old clothes as you get smaller so you don't get tempted to eat bad again and have the clothes there and ready, keeping a few around to use as a measure can be a great way to track your progress.

Use the Scale

Another way that you can measure and track the amount of progress that you make while intermittent fasting is to use the scale. This helps you to see exactly how much weight you have lost and how far you have gone since you first got started. The reason that it is so far down on the list is that it isn't always the best indicator.

Sure, you do want to see your weight go down. This helps you to fight off many health conditions and shows that you are healthier and more fit overall. But if you are adding in exercise, especially strength training, you may find that the numbers don't always add up the right way. Muscle weighs more than fat so while you are burning fat with your fast, you may be building up muscle, and that can give you a higher number on the scale. Use the scale as a tool, but make sure that it is used as a complement to the other methods we discuss here.

Chapter 18: Should I Add Any Exercise into My Fast?

The most effective intermittent fast is one where you add lots of healthy exercises as well. Intermittent fasting can do a great deal of good when it comes to cutting calories and helping you lose weight, but the other part of the equation is for you to add in some exercise as well. Exercise can help you maintain your muscle mass, burn more calories than fasting alone and give you more energy to get through the day.

A common question that people on an intermittent fast may have is how they can add in more exercise to their day and which exercises are the best. To keep it simple, any exercise that you enjoy doing and that you will keep doing for the long term is going to be perfect. However, there are times when a specific workout will be more effective or enjoyable to you.

If you can, it is best to do a good mixture of workouts with some weight training, cardio, and strength training mixed together. But doing one type of exercise that you love is better than not doing anything at all. Let's explore some of the different types of workouts that you can consider with intermittent fasting, and how to do them safely to get the best results.

Weight Lifting and Intermittent Fasting

When it comes to intermittent fasting, many people like to begin a weight lifting or strength training workout. This can be beneficial in several ways. First, it helps you to build up lots of lean and strong muscles that make you look trimmer and can burn through more fat and calories than just intermittent fasting alone. Strength training can also work when you are in a fasted state because you don't need to burn up fuel as quickly as you do with cardio.

Many people who add weight training to their routine will do it while they are in their fasted state, although it is fine to add in anywhere you have time. Doing this during the fasted state can help you burn through even more glycogen than before, giving you better results.

If you do choose to weight train during a fast, try to set it up so that you end your fasting window right after the exercise is done. This way, you can get the benefits of training while fasted, but then you can provide the body with the nutrients it needs to repair those muscles once the workout is done.

With weight training and intermittent fasting, fewer reps with more weight are the best option. This helps you to get the stronger muscle that looks lean, without having to spend hours in the gym. Start out small, and perhaps even skip the workouts in the beginning. You will get stronger and will be able to take on more weight but remember that this is a time when your body is adjusting, and you never want to overdo it.

Is HIIT a Good Idea to Add into My Exercise Plan

One thing that you may want to consider adding into your exercise program is HIIT or high-intensity interval training. This type of exercise can really help add in many extra health benefits, and it doesn't require you spending hours in the gym like other methods.

Researchers have taken time to look at HIIT exercises and found that they can be effective. It has been shown that doing three rounds of 20 seconds of HIIT three times a week can give the body as many benefits as you get while running on the treadmill. Instead of spending all that time running on the treadmill or at the gym, you could spend about ten to 15 minutes on your workout and get the same benefits.

For those who are just getting started on their own intermittent fast and aren't used to the effects, or those who aren't used to doing a lot of working out, it can be great news to help them get started. You will get a ton of benefits with just a short burst of exercise, and who wouldn't want to see that?

You get some choices when it comes to HIIT. You can either make the whole workout based on this idea or find ways to add it into your regular workout. For example, you can either do ten minutes of the spurts or go out for a two-mile walk and add in three or four rounds with a sprint that lasts about 20 seconds each. Both will provide you with good benefits to your health in a shorter amount of time.

Do I Need to Worry About Preserving My Muscles During an Intermittent Fast?

Many experts agree that out of the health benefits that you get out of exercise and diet, 80 percent comes from your diet. The other 20 percent will come from the exercise that you do. This means that it is more important to concentrate on consuming the right kinds of foods to help you lose weight and keep your muscle strength intact. However, adding exercise to the mixture can really help you get healthier as well.

Some research looked at the data of participants who were on the show *The Biggest Loser*. The information that was looked at for this research included the resting metabolic rate, the total amount of energy used, and the total body fat of all the participants and these numbers were measured three times. They were measured right when the program began, after six weeks into the program, and then finally done after 30 weeks.

Researchers found that the diet the participants consumed was the most responsible for the weight that they lost. And only about 65 percent of that loss in weight came from body fat. The rest came from a loss in lean muscle mass. Exercise alone resulted in an only fat loss with a slight increase in lean muscle mass. This means that it is possible to lose a little bit of muscle mass with just diet alone but adding in exercise will ensure that you can maintain and even grow that muscle mass while eating a healthy diet like on an intermittent fast.

Chapter 19: What If I'm Not Seeing Results from My Fast?

An intermittent fast is a great way for you to get in the best health of your life and lose weight all at the same time. However, there are times when you may not be seeing the exact results that you want. When this happens, many fasters ask why they aren't losing weight. There is usually a pretty simple explanation for this. The most common one is that you have lost some weight, but because of increased muscle tone, or the natural variations that occur in the weight of your body through the day, it isn't showing up on the scale. There are several reasons why you may not be seeing the results of your intermittent fast right away, and some of these are:

•*How long have you been on the intermittent fast?*

The amount of time that you have been on the intermittent fast can make a difference. If you just got started with fasting, you are not going to see a ton of weight loss in just a week. It will take a bit of time for your body to adapt to this new eating plan. While many people who go on a fast see results in weight loss right away, this early loss can often be because there are changes in the amount of water the body holds onto.

This means that one of the reasons that you don't see much weight loss is because you didn't lose a lot of water in the beginning. Even using a tape measure to check your waist and other parts of the body, it may be a little bit slow to show the differences that are occurring based on where you lose the fat.

If you have been on the fast for a long time and you have stopped losing weight, or it seems like you are hitting a plateau, several things could be to blame here. These can include:

oIf you are having weight loss, but it is slow, the actual weight that is lost can be hidden by many other natural variations that we go through each day. Our weight can vary by about two pounds up or down due to the way that the body holds onto water or the foods that are passing through our system. If you were losing weight and then it seems to stop, it could be because of some of the variations that happen in your body. You may be holding onto water more or even gaining some muscle.

oSecond, as you start to lose weight, the body is going to need less energy to survive, so the speed of weight loss is going to slow down, and it may even plateau. To help make more progress, you will need to make efforts to use more energy each day by increasing your levels of activity. Combine this with a reduction in the number of calories that you take in each day. Any time that you stall in your weight loss, consider recalculating your daily energy needs to see if you need to change it up.

oThird, as you get comfortable with the intermittent fast, it is sometimes easy to let things slip a little, and you may not be as strict about your calorie intake on the fasting days or the length of your fast. This loss of focus can be a reason that you are not losing weight any longer or a reason why you have stalled out.

If any of these are true with you, it is important just to keep calm and wait it out for a bit. You may need to wait a few weeks to find out if you really plateaued or not. In the meantime, recalculate the energy that you expend during the day and check that you are not eating more calories or cutting into your fast earlier than you think. If nothing is working, it may be time to upgrade to a different version of the fast, such as going from the 5:2 diet to the alternate day fast.

•How much and how quickly do you want to lose weight?

If you are at a pretty healthy weight and you don't need to lose much, then you will find that the rate at which you lose weight is going to be a lot slower compared to someone who has quite a bit to lose. If you are already close to your healthy weight range and you are in shape, and you are trying to lose a few pounds in just a week or two, then you may end up being disappointed in this process. Intermittent fasting can still work, but you must realize that it is going to take more time for those who are closer to their ideal and healthy weight range.

As you start to carry around less fat, your body is going to slow the weight loss through several different methods. Although scientists are still in debate about whether our bodies have a preferred set weight at which weight loss efforts are going to stall, in practice, many people have this problem. If you are already at a pretty healthy weight for you, then it may be time to consider whether you need to make some revisions to your target when it comes to weight loss.

If you still want to lose some weight, or you have a lot of weight to lose, and you get stalled, then it is possible that some medical issues are the reason behind this struggle. Some conditions like fibromyalgia, PCOS, and thyroid problems can all make it difficult for you to lose the weight that you would like.

The best thing that you can do is think about the amount that you need to lose to help make yourself healthier rather than giving yourself a target that is hard to reach. You also need to accept that weight loss can be a very slow process since intermittent fasting is all about changing your lifestyle for the better. Intermittent fasting is not just a fad that you try for a few weeks; it is something that you stick with for the long haul, even if that means you don't lose weight as quickly as you want.

Since this type of eating is more about sticking to it for the long term, it may be time to consider whether a change to your method of fasting is the way that would help you lose weight quicker. Changing things up on occasion can keep you from getting bored with your version of intermittent fasting and could help to shorten your eating window, so it is easier to lose weight. Why not try out the alternate day fast for a few weeks or change up your eating, so you take in fewer carbs? These simple changes to the fast can make a big difference in how much you enjoy the fast and even the amount that you can lose.

- *Are you eating too much during your eating window or eating the wrong types of foods?*

Another reason why you may not be losing weight is that you are overeating during your non-fasting times. While intermittent fasting can help you to reduce your caloric intake, it is not a cure-all, and it is still possible for an individual to eat too much during their non-fasting periods.

The first thing to consider, if you lost a lot of weight, is that you might need to take in even less food to sustain your body. If it's been a while since you went through and figured out how many calories you need to consume, then now is the time to do it again. You may find that you are inadvertently taking in more calories than your body needs, and it is time to cut it down a little bit more.

In some cases, you may be doing well on a fast, and then suddenly, the days when you are super hungry start to happen more frequently. Intermittent fasting can help to control the appetite, but sometimes, those extra hungry days are going to start getting out of hand. When this happens, it may be time to add in an extra fast day to your schedule, or at least extending the length of your fasting period to help get that appetite back under control.

If you are suffering from insulin resistance, be aware that your body is going to be very sensitive to any carbs that you take in, especially refined carbs and sugars. Carbs are going to stimulate the body to release insulin, which makes it hard for you to burn any of your stored fat. And for some people, once they take in a few carbs, they get into a cycle of being hungry and having a lot of cravings at the same time.

If this sounds like something that happens to you, it may be time to consider changing the type of diet you are on. Most people are just fine sticking with a diet that allows some whole grains and other carbs, but for those who are sensitive to them and who seem to have trouble on their fast, it may be time to go on a low carb diet. With this kind of diet, you will avoid all carbs on your fast days and then severely reduce carbs on your non-fasting times. This may seem extreme, but you will be amazed at how much it can help when you are struggling with keeping your calories in check with an intermittent fast.

Before we end, a word about alcohol while fasting. Some people find that drinking alcohol can slow down the amount of weight they can lose while also increasing their appetite on those non-fast days. This substance can also make it hard on fasting days. This is because alcohol is going to influence how the body can handle carbs, and this particularly affects the liver. If you do drink while you are fasting, it may be time to consider cutting down on how much alcohol you consume. You don't have to give it up completely but be careful and make sure that you reduce or eliminate it the day before one of your fasts to get the best results.

Intermittent fasting can be a fun way to help you lose weight and get in the best shape of your life. However, there are also times when you will hit a plateau and can't seem to lose any more weight, despite following all the same steps that you did in the past. When this happens to you, it can be really frustrating, and you want to figure out how to make it change. Follow some of the tips that are in this chapter, and it won't be long before your weight loss begins to happen again!

Conclusion

Thanks for making it through to the end of *Intermittent Fasting: How to Lose Weight, Burn Fat, and Increase*

is the right eating protocol for you to follow. This eating plan will provide you with a ton of great benefits and *Mental Clarity without Having to Give up All Your Favorite Foods*. It should have been informative and provided you with all the tools needed to achieve your goals whatever they may be.

The next step is to decide if intermittent fasting can easily help you lose weight while not feeling deprived in the process. And with the different methods that are available with intermittent fasting, it is something you will really enjoy and can easily fit into your daily schedule without much hassle.

Inside this guidebook, we looked at an intermittent fast and how it can be so much more effective than your current eating plan. With the current American diet, we are taking in too many calories and getting into a horrible cycle that makes us sick. The body may crave those bad foods because they provide it with an easy and constant source of fuel, but we are slowly setting ourselves up for a whole bunch of chronic illnesses.

Intermittent fasting helps us to change all that. It allows us the option to cut down on how many calories we consume during the day while also naturally speeding up the metabolism. Add in there that you will not give the body a constant source of glucose any longer, so it must rely on stored glycogen and other resources. It is no wonder that intermittent fasting can help solve health problems while also helping us lose weight.

We also looked at some of the basics that come with intermittent fasting, how to get started, the different health benefits you can get from fasting, the steps that you can follow to get the most out of this fasting method, the side effects that you may notice when you first get started, the things that you can do if fasting doesn't seem to be working right for you and how to fix these issues, and so much more.

While there may be many different eating and diet plans out there, intermittent fasting is one that seems to work well for so many people. It helps them learn how to listen to their body, how to eat more healthily, and how to allow their body to get into fat burning mode all on its own.

If you enjoyed this book, a review on Amazon would be greatly appreciated.

Thanks for your support!

Part 2: Keto Diet

The Ultimate Ketogenic Diet Guide for Weight Loss and Mental Clarity, Including How to Get into Ketosis, a 21-Day Meal Plan, Keto Fasting Tips for Beginners and Meal Prep Ideas

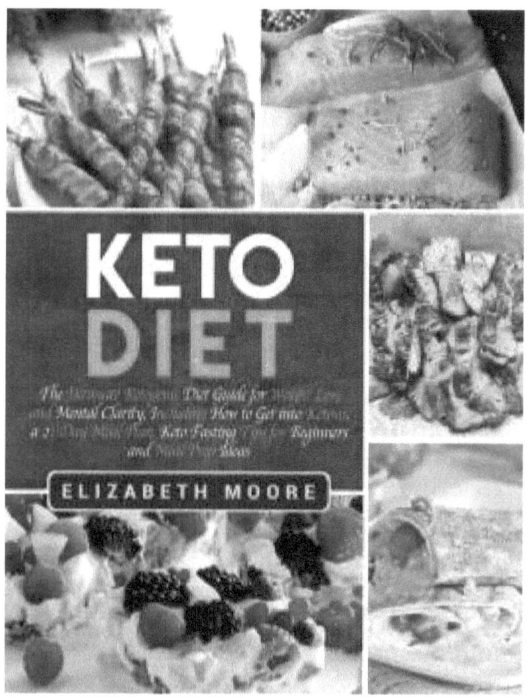

Introduction

The standard ketogenic diet has been around for nearly a century. Unlike the fad diets that fade in and out of popularity, the ketogenic diet has remained due to its amazing health benefits. However, the weight loss benefits of the ketogenic diet have recently been discovered by the masses, making it not only a wonderful choice for those with neurological illnesses, but for people who want to lose weight or live a healthy lifestyle, as well.

In this book, you will learn what makes the ketogenic diet different and special, the science behind why the ketogenic diet works, tips, and tricks to help you along on your journey, how to pair a healthful ketogenic diet with exercise to maximize results, a twenty-one-day meal plan, and much more!

Whether your weight goals are to get a killer beach body, a slim look for the holidays, or general health and well-being, the ketogenic diet has been shown both scientifically and through personal experience to greatly reduce body fat. Even if you are someone who lives with a disease that may cause obesity, such as polycystic ovary syndrome, the ketogenic diet has been shown to help reduce weight. Specifically, the ketogenic diet targets that pesky fat around the abdomen, which not only makes finding clothing difficult but also is the most dangerous and disease-promoting type of fat.

Whether you want to use the ketogenic diet to lose weight, gain weight, improve your health, protect against neurodegenerative diseases, or to aid in the treatment of a loved one, then you can find what you are looking for with this unique high-fat and low-carbohydrate lifestyle.

Chapter 1: What is the Ketogenic Diet?

To put it simply, the ketogenic is a low-carb and high-fat diet in which you consume moderate amounts of protein. Yet there is more to it than that. Firstly, the ketogenic diet is different from other low-carbohydrate diets, which often contain an average of twenty-five to fifty grams of carbohydrates, more than is allowed on keto. In this chapter, you will learn all of the basic must-learn knowledge about this incredible diet and lifestyle.

This chapter is not about the century-old history of the ketogenic diet, although the ketogenic diet was established nearly one-hundred years ago in the treatment of epilepsy. Since that time, it has been shown to treat drug-resistant epilepsy and other neurodegenerative and neurological illnesses. In recent years, due to the successful healing from the ketogenic diet, more people have learned of this powerful plan and soon found it to be an amazing weight loss option. Yet, if you are someone who is underweight or at your ideal weight, you can also gain or maintain weight on this diet – if that is what your body needs and your doctor recommends.

The Essential Mitochondrial Cells

Every living organism, whether animal or plant, is composed of many important cells that are microscopic compartments that are found in the membrane. While cells themselves are microscopic, they contain even smaller sub-compartments inside of them. These sub-compartments are known as "organelles" and contribute to many essential functions for the cell's survival. One amazing aspect of our cells is that they are the smallest thing in nature that can reproduce themselves.

The mitochondria are an aspect of many of our cells, also known as a powerhouse. The cells that contain mitochondria can convert protein, carbohydrates, and fat into energy for the body's survival.

The mitochondria organelles are found in every human and animal and are utilized to produce ninety percent of the energy that is required for survival. Without the mitochondrial cells, we would be unable to live. Yet these cells do not only keep us alive, but they also aid in breaking down waste, recycling waste, and produce necessary chemicals.

The mitochondria have an important role in preventing tumor growth and cancer and are even targeted in some anti-cancer drugs because of this. This is because the mitochondria can cause old cells, which could become dangerous components of tumors, to die and decompose. This allows new healthy cells to grow in their place.

The mitochondria use a process called "oxidative phosphorylation" to effectively convert the food you consume into energy needed to survive and support the brain and organs. Yet this process requires a lot of oxygen, and if there is not enough, the mitochondrial cells will be unable to function. This means that when a person has a stroke or a heart attack, the oxygen is restricted in either the brain or the heart. The lack of oxygen in these important organs prevents the mitochondria from converting energy, leading to cell damage or even death. Even if the oxygen returns to the area, the quick return will cause the cells to be overwhelmed, triggering the production of cancer-causing free radicals.

While the mitochondrial cells can use either fat, carbohydrates, or protein for fuel, it will prioritize carbohydrates. This means that anytime you eat sugar, potatoes, grains, or anything else that contains carbohydrates the mitochondrial cells will convert them before any of the protein or fat.

There are multiple reasons as to why the mitochondria prefer the carbohydrates, and therefore glucose.

Firstly, because carbohydrates can be converted into energy more quickly than either of the other fuels, and secondly, the body is only capable of storing limited quantities of carbohydrates. After the carbohydrates are converted into glucose, it is stored in the liver and muscles. The remaining amount of glucose must be transmuted into lipids (fat) and stored as body fat. Therefore, in order to prevent from needing to convert the glucose into lipids, and to get the quickest form of energy possible, the mitochondria make use of the glucose before other fuels. This may not seem like a negative, but glucose is not the most efficient fuel source.

Fats, also known as lipids, are the most efficient source of energy. Not only that, but the human body is unable to produce healthy fats such as linoleic acid on its own, making fats an essential portion of the human diet – unlike carbohydrates, which the body can function and thrive without. A few of the necessary functions of dietary fat is helping the blood clot in a healthy manner, aiding in brain development, and controlling the levels of inflammation.

While fats may take longer to digest, we are enabled with many bodily functions which help us healthily process them. For instance, under our tongue, we have a gland which will release the enzyme lingual lipase, which then splits the molecules in the fat. After we swallow the fats and they eventually arrive in the stomach, they are further digested by being combined with gastric lipase, constantly being churned together with the muscles of the stomach. Once the process is complete, the globules of the fat are emulsified and transformed from large to small.

Once the lipids depart the stomach, they reach the small intestines and continue to be emulsified with bile that is released from the gallbladder, specifically for this purpose. Once they are broken down into even smaller molecules that can be absorbed into the lining of the intestines, they travel to the liver and are turned into energy.

While this is the digestion process for most fats, there are exceptions. While commonly fats that people consume are a long-chain triglyceride, which requires a long process to be transmuted into a smaller triglyceride, this is not true of all fats. Some fats are medium-chain triglycerides – these are especially common in coconut oil. These fats are digested much quicker and can be absorbed by the liver to use as energy right away.

Protein, like fat, is another essential nutrient and energy source. Whether the protein is from animal products or plant-based products, after arriving in the stomach, it is broken down with acids and enzymes until the molecules are small enough to reach the small intestines. On their arrival, they are further broken down with the help of gastric juice from the liver and pancreas. This process converts the protein into an amino acid. The amino acid can then be absorbed into the bloodstream where it is used to repair cells and provide energy.

Through a process of greatly restricting carbohydrates, the ketogenic diet can strong-arm the mitochondria into using more optimal sources of fuel, meaning fat, and what is known as ketones.

While some of our cells, such as our red blood cells, kidney medulla, testicle cells, and brain cells may require glucose, they will not be deprived. Only ten percent of our cells require glucose, and in the absence of dietary glucose, this can be provided through the process of gluconeogenesis.

This amazing process of gluconeogenesis can transmute amino acids, glycerol, and lactate into the needed amount of glucose for these cells. Yet it does this without overproducing glucose; therefore, it will not interfere with the ketogenic diet.

Although, it is important to provide your body with enough protein, therefore amino acids, to be converted into glucose. Otherwise, your body could convert up to 2.2 pounds of your lean muscle mass daily. Thankfully, with moderate levels of protein, you should not encounter any problems.

The ketone bodies that are produced on the ketogenic diet can be used as a new type of energy source. Once the body is consuming an extremely low carbohydrate diet, then the liver creates ketones. This process can also help take the burden off of the gluconeogenesis process, requiring to convert five times fewer amino acids than it otherwise would need, since the ketones can often be used in place of glucose.

This is especially helpful because while the brain does require a fast-acting fuel source, such as glucose, this causes it to create reactive oxygen species, which are an extremely dangerous and a damaging type of oxidant. Yet up to seventy-five percent of the brain contains the ability to use ketones for fuel rather than glucose. This not only reduces oxidative stress, and therefore, your risk of cancer, but it can also lessen your risk of age-related diseases and other illnesses.

Along with being produced when on a low carbohydrate diet, ketones are also produced when we are fasting, or in the worst case, starving. Thankfully, on the ketogenic diet, we can receive all of the benefits provided with ketones while still providing our bodies with all of the health and necessary nutrients it needs. To produce the ketones after glucose is depleted from the body, the fat you have eaten, and your body fat, is released into the bloodstream. Afterward, these molecules are broken down with the process of beta-oxidation, which will allow the cells that do not contain mitochondria to use them as an energy source. After the beta-oxidation process converts the lipid cells into acetyl-CoA, then they are once again converted, this time into citrate. This can then be turned into GTP, ATP, and ketones.

While often referred to as 'ketone bodies', scientifically, they are not technically classified as bodies, but rather they are a water-soluble substance that comes in three forms: acetone, acetoacetate, and beta-hydroxybutyrate. They are then released into the bloodstream where they may be used as an energy source by the mitochondria. This is especially effective because, unlike fatty acids, ketones can cross the blood-brain barrier and be used for the brain and nervous system. Not only does this help prevent the development of neurodegenerative disorders, but it has even been shown to aid in the healing of traumatic brain injuries.

What are some of the other benefits of using ketones as a fuel source?

• Ketones are a more efficient energy source and require much less oxygen to process. This increases brain energy, clarity, and decreases aging of the brain.

• The brain may sometimes develop an excess of glutamate, causing it to become an excitotoxin and damage our nerve cells, eventually leading to neurodegenerative diseases. While glutamate is important and essential for neural function, memory formation, communication, and learning, it is also important to have an inhibitory transmitter to keep the amount of glutamate balanced. Thankfully, ketones increase the amount of GABA, which will naturally help regulate the amount of glutamate by inhibiting an excess of this neurotransmitter. This process may help in preventing Alzheimer's disease, multiple sclerosis, Parkinson's disease, and Lou Gehrig's disease.

• Ketones, as well as the healthy fats on the ketogenic diet, have been shown to decrease inflammation. Not only can this aid in the treatment of chronic disease, but it can even reduce inflammation in the brain, helping us age better, and reduce the risk of neurological illness.

• The longer you are in a state of ketosis, meaning producing ketones, the more your body will produce neural mitochondrial cells, as well as increasing their effectiveness. This is amazing since the mitochondrial cells are the ones needed to utilize any fuel source. Therefore, more of the brain will have the ability to use fats as fuel, providing many great health benefits.

• While most of the neurons in the brain are formed before birth, there are specific areas of the brain which remain able to produce new neurons from stem cells. This process, neurogenesis, can be stimulated by the BDNF protein and is increased by the production of ketones. This process promotes the growth of neurons and synapses, especially improving the health of the hippocampus, cortex, and forebrain.

The Macro Ratio

The macro ratio is extremely important on the ketogenic diet because without it you are unlikely to stay in the ketosis process, where your body uses fat and ketones for fuel. This ratio is the amount of the main nutrients you need, meaning carbohydrates, fat, and protein. If you do not eat the correct amount of these, you are likely to eat too many carbohydrates and too little protein.

When keeping track of your carbohydrate intake on the ketogenic diet, it is important to track the "net" carbohydrates and not the "total" carbohydrates. This is because net carbohydrates have the indigestible carbs from the equation. This means that both fiber and most sugar alcohols are removed.

While sugar alcohols are a safe and natural sweetener option, it is advised to be cautious. Certain types of sugar alcohol, such as maltitol, are more likely to cause stomach upset. Whereas, erythritol is much gentler on the stomach and can be eaten in larger amounts. Yet you still need to be careful not to over-consume sugar alcohols of any type; otherwise, you may develop diarrhea. Another reason maltitol is not advised is that, unlike most sugar alcohols, it does cause a spike in blood sugar and alcohol, not really making it ketogenic friendly. Thankfully, maltitol is no longer a common sweetener and most foods that are sweetened with sugar alcohol, such as certain brands of zero calorie soda, use erythritol and sometimes combine it with stevia leaf extract.

It is important to eat plenty of low-carbohydrate vegetables on the ketogenic diet, both for nutrients and fiber. Not only does a high fiber content aid in preventing constipation, but it can also lower your risk of disease and increase absorption of vital nutrients.

On the ketogenic diet, carbohydrates will be the most limited, mostly to non-starchy vegetables and low-sugar fruits. The fruits that are ideal are avocados and olives (yes, they are fruits) and small servings of berries. Melon may also be eaten on occasion, but only in small servings.

While most people may not think of nuts as being a carbohydrate-rich food, they can be surprisingly high. For this reason, cashews and pistachios are a no-go. Although, in moderation, macadamia nuts, pecans, and almonds can be a wonderful option. Peanuts are debated on the ketogenic diet, so it is up to you – just watch your serving size.

While whole grains and beans might be high in fiber, and therefore lower in net carbohydrates than their processed counterparts, they are still high in carbohydrates either way and should be avoided completely on the ketogenic diet. The only exception is low-carbohydrate soybean products such as tofu.

On the ketogenic diet, you should be calculating how many net carbohydrates you are eating. The number one mistake people make is not tracking this, which either kicks them out of ketosis or prevents weight loss. The standard number of net carbohydrates is twenty-five to thirty grams, yet some people go extremely hardcore keto with only twelve or less net carbs a day.

The intake of fat is the core of the ketogenic diet. This is where you will get a majority of your calories from, and many nutrients and health-promoting properties as well. The amount of fat you will require varies from person to person, depending on their weight goals. If someone's goal is to lose weight, they may eat a small calorie deficit, or if their goal is to gain weight, they can greatly increase their caloric intake. While you don't have to worry about too many fats kicking you out of ketosis, such as too many carbohydrates can, it is still important to track the number of fats you are eating. This is because fat is extremely high in calories, and if you are not tracking how much you are eating, you may easily eat six to a hundred extra calories in fat. In fact, this is the most common cause for a lack of weight loss, so track your macros!

When consuming fats on the ketogenic diet, you are not just consuming any fat – you can't go around eating random fried foods that happen to be low-carbohydrate. Avoid trans fats, and limit saturated fats to coconut oil. While some saturated fats may not be the best for you, study after study has proven the health benefits of coconut oil and its ability to aid in healing and weight loss. In general, you want to avoid vegetable oils such as corn and soy. Rather, use fruit, seed, and nut oils, such as avocado, olive, sesame, and macadamia. When consuming butter, try to use grass-fed when possible, as it has an astounding amount of more health-promoting qualities and nutrients than grain-fed butter.

When beginning the ketogenic diet, you need to use an online calculator to find your own macro ratio. This will tell you the exact amount of carbohydrates, fats, and proteins you should eat depending on your weight, activity levels, and goals. This is important not only to keep you in ketosis and help you reach your weight goals but to help you do so in a healthy manner.

What many people don't realize is that if you are not eating enough protein on a low-carbohydrate diet, your body will go into a process of gluconeogenesis, where your body will begin to convert your lean muscle tone into fuel. This is obviously unhealthy and undesirable;

therefore, it is important to eat enough protein to prevent muscle atrophy. In general, you want twenty-five percent of your day's calories to come from protein. The easiest sources of protein are meats, fish, shellfish, eggs, and whole-fat dairy products, though tofu is also low in carbohydrates and is great for vegetarians or vegans.

In a nutshell, your individual macro ratio is calculated with your recommended daily caloric intake, depending on your weight and activity level. A minimum of twenty percent protein and the ideal of twenty-five percent protein of your caloric intake is recommended. You can consume no more than thirty grams of net carbohydrates, and the remaining portion of your caloric intake is made up of healthy fats.

The Types of Ketogenic Diets

The proportions of the macro ratio mentioned above are for the traditional ketogenic diet. Along with vegan, vegetarian, and dairy-free ketogenic diets, there are two additional types of ketogenic diets. These are especially wonderful for people who are highly active.

The Targeted Ketogenic Diet is a great option for people who are highly active or athletes who require a higher carbohydrate level. This option is best for people who work out irregularly or only workout at high intensities twice a week. Thankfully, light and moderate exercises, such as yoga or jogging, require no extra carbohydrates. If you are someone who uses HIIT training, weightlifting, or regular high-intensity sports, then the targeted ketogenic diet may be for you.

In order to follow the targeted ketogenic diet simply consume between twenty-five to fifty net carbohydrates thirty minutes prior to a high-intensity workout. You want to ensure that you do not eat too many carbohydrates, as you want to have to ability to burn them off during the workout so that you can stay in ketosis. Keep your carbohydrate intake limited to healthy sources, such as fruits and vegetables; sweet potatoes and beets are wonderful health-promoting options.

If you are attempting to lose weight, then be sure to include the calories from the carbohydrates into your daily caloric goal.

Unlike the targeted ketogenic diet, the Cyclical Ketogenic Diet is for people who work out regularly. It is extremely important to have a set workout schedule where you work out at least three times a week, preferably four or five days a week. Otherwise, you will be unable to go into a state of ketosis.

Unlike on the targeted ketogenic diet, where you are only consuming carbohydrates directly before a workout, on the cyclical version you have a day or two where you load up on high-carbohydrate foods. This is why a regular, consistent, and high-intensity schedule is needed for this version of the ketogenic diet. The proportions are different on the cyclical ketogenic diet, and are as follows:

Day One: In order to prepare an anabolic state in which you can heal and build muscle, begin the first day by consuming a high-carbohydrate meal five hours prior to an intense workout. Then, two hours before the workout, eat a small carbohydrate snack, of about twenty-five to fifty net carbohydrates. Fruit is a great choice, as it has both glucose and fructose, which can help refill the liver's glycogen.

You want about seventy percent of your day's calories to be from carbohydrates, fifteen percent to be from protein, and fifteen percent to be from fats.

Day Two: On the second day of the cyclical ketogenic diet, lower your carbohydrate intake slightly, so that it makes up sixty percent of your caloric intake. Twenty-five percent of the caloric intake should be protein, and fifteen percent should be fat. It is important that you take a day of rest. Some people who work out regularly don't take rest days, and this is a drain on your body and unproductive. In fact, rest days are an incredibly important aspect of exercise that allows your muscles to heal and grow back stronger. You are unable to reach your full potential without rest. After six in the evening try to avoid eating, as you want to have a short fast until breakfast, to help yourself go back into ketosis as soon as possible.

Day Three: On the third day, to help burn off the carbohydrates from the fuel-up days, you want to work out on an empty stomach. In fact, try to work out on an empty stomach every day. This process will also promote fat loss. Keep your carbohydrate count no higher than ten net carbohydrates.

Day Four: Take a break from the high-intensity workout by doing a medium-intensity workout on the fourth day. On this day, you can consume between fifteen and twenty net carbohydrates.

Days Five and Six: Continue with the standard ketogenic diet and your regular high-intensity workout.

Day Seven: Day of recuperation and rest.

Day Eight: Day of regular high-intensity or medium-intensity workout.

Remember, this method is only for people who have a regular high-intensity workout schedule.

The Micro Nutrients

The second biggest mistake people make on the ketogenic diet, along with not tracking their macronutrients, is not consuming enough micronutrients. These nutrients are the vitamins and minerals you need in smaller amounts, such as magnesium, vitamin C, and folate. It is essential to get these vitamins in low-carbohydrate vegetables and fruits, but they can also be found in grass-fed meats, grass-fed butter, eggs, and organ meats, such as the liver. Following is a list of some of the most important micronutrients to ensure that you do not become deficient on the ketogenic diet:

Sodium

Some of the most important micronutrients to ensure you get enough of are electrolytes. One of these electrolytes, sodium, is largely avoided due to the negative attention it receives for heart health. Yet a deficiency in sodium also has a negative impact on your heart; therefore, it is important to retain a balanced sodium intake. Remember: on the ketogenic diet you will not be eating highly processed foods that are high in sodium. Also, when you begin the process of ketosis, your body will flush itself of excess fluids, resulting in a loss of electrolytes. It is imperative to refuel on both water and electrolytes, including sodium.

People may also become more inclined to sodium deficiencies as they lose weight. This is because people develop a healthier insulin response as they lose weight, and as they become less insulin resistant, their body will hold onto less sodium. This is especially true if you are maintaining an active lifestyle or in the heat and sweating more.

If you suspect you may have a sodium deficiency, watch for symptoms of headaches, fatigue, and weakness. This is especially important during the beginning weeks of the ketogenic diet when you are losing mostly water weight. Doctors regularly recommend consuming between three to five grams of sodium daily.

While you can simply salt your food more, drinking low-carbohydrate and sugar-free electrolyte drinks can help keep your sodium and other electrolyte levels up. If you suspect your symptoms may be from electrolyte imbalance, then try drinking one of these drinks, such as Ultima Replenisher, and see if your symptoms improve.

Potassium

Another essential micronutrient is potassium, and a deficiency may include symptoms of irritability, constipation, weakness, muscle loss, irregular heartbeat, palpitations, and skin disorders. In severe cases, it may even lead to heart failure. In order to prevent deficiencies, it is recommended to consume about forty-five-hundred milligrams of potassium daily.

Some high sources of potassium include mushrooms, kale, and avocado. Spinach is also high in potassium, but the oxalates in spinach block the absorption making it nearly useless.

Magnesium

Magnesium impacts over three-hundred of our biochemical functions, which can affect our cell reproduction, energy, the formation of fatty acids, and protein synthesis. Symptoms of a sodium deficiency may include muscle cramps, dizziness, and fatigue. It is recommended to consume an average of five-hundred milligrams a day.

Some great sources of magnesium include Swiss chard, oysters, and pumpkin seeds.

Calcium

The fourth of the electrolytes, calcium, is essential for controlling the clotting of blood, regulating blood pressure, strengthening bones and teeth, and transmitting signals between nerve cells. To consume enough calcium to prevent deficiency, try to consume between one and two grams per day.

Some foods high in calcium include cheddar cheese, sardines, raw broccoli, cooked kale, and almonds.

Iron

While spinach is infamous for being high in iron, it contains oxalates which block it from being absorbed. Rather than spinach, try raising your iron levels with mushrooms, olives, nuts, seeds, dark leafy greens, eggs, meat, and coconut milk.

There are two types of iron, and both are absorbed differently. While plants can be high in the non-heme type of iron, this is often not easily absorbed. Therefore, when consuming iron, try to consume it in small amounts throughout the day, as it is better absorbed in small doses. Other ways you can boost absorption is by cooking in cast iron pans. Iron can also be more easily absorbed when your iron stores are low, and less is absorbed when they are high. Eating vitamin C with spinach may increase the absorption rate by five times.

Try to avoid consuming coffee, tea, and chocolate within two hours of eating iron-rich foods, as they contain compounds that block the absorption of this important nutrient. The recommended dosage of iron for adults is 8.7 milligrams, though people who menstruate should try to consume 14.8 milligrams a day to prevent anemia. Obviously, it is best to discuss this with your doctor in case you have low or high levels of iron.

Vitamin D3

While the ketogenic diet does not cause a predisposition to this important vitamin, known as the sunshine vitamin, many people already have a deficiency regardless of their diet. Yet this vitamin is vital for the immune system, bone health, muscle function, and nerve function. It also aids in protecting against illnesses such as depression, heart disease, diabetes, autoimmune disease, and cancer. This important vitamin even helps promote the absorption of calcium and phosphate.

We can absorb vitamin D3 into the skin through exposure to sunlight, but due to the risks of skin cancer, this can also be dangerous in large amounts. Therefore, many doctors recommend for people to take a daily D3 vitamin.

The Safety of the Ketogenic Diet

People may raise concerns over the ketogenic diet and its safety, but time and time again it has been proven to be safe in healthy individuals, and even in many people with chronic illnesses. Obviously, if you have a chronic illness or disease, you should first consult with your doctor before making any dietary changes.

While one of the prime goals when on the ketogenic diet is to produce ketone bodies for fuel and brain health, some people may worry about a condition known as ketoacidosis. This may be caused when a person is deficient in insulin, which causes the liver to overproduce ketones at a rate the body is unable to handle. This serious condition is dangerous and can be caused by uncontrolled type I or type II diabetes.

With both types of diabetes, it is caused when there is too little insulin to communicate with the cells to let them know that they have enough energy. This deficiency then causes the fat and liver cells to enter starvation mode, even after eating a full meal. Due to this, the fat cells begin to release too many triglycerides into the bloodstream in order to provide more energy and fuel. The liver then uses this to create ketones, but it creates much more than the body can handle.

This process causes high blood sugar and a buildup of ketones in the bloodstream, which results in water being dumped from the body and causing the blood to turn acidic. Between the low insulin, high ketones, and low fluids, the acidic blood, known as metabolic acidosis, prevents the body from properly functioning.

While this condition is extremely dangerous and you should seek medical attention immediately, thankfully it is preventable. Studies have shown that on the ketogenic diet people with diabetes can have much more healthy levels of blood sugar and prevent insulin resistance, which should prevent ketoacidosis. The ketogenic diet has even been shown to help people with diabetes go off of their prescribed medicines with the guidance of their prescribing physician.

Some other good news is that people without diabetes are unlikely ever to develop ketoacidosis and that the ketogenic diet has not been shown to cause this condition. Even better is that eating a healthy diet, such as the ketogenic diet, may prevent you from ever developing diabetes in the future.

While the ketogenic diet is generally safe for most people, it is not recommended for people with kidney disease. Likewise, it has not been tested on people who are pregnant or breastfeeding, making it not recommended for these people until further studies are conducted.

Chapter 2: Why Choose the Keto Lifestyle

There are many benefits to the ketogenic diet, including increased energy, weight loss, and both the treatment and prevention of many diseases. In this chapter, we will go over some of the most common reasons to choose the ketogenic diet and the health-promoting qualities it may provide.

Weight Loss

While science has shown that BMI has little merit and you can be both fat and healthy, and there is no shame in being fat and proud even if you are unhealthy, there is still much scientific backing showing that having a higher body fat percentage increases your risk of disease. Many people may try crash diets to lower their weight, but years of these diets not only take a toll on your health but lower your metabolism and make it more difficult to lose weight over time. You often even gain the weight back soon after quitting the diet.

Thankfully, the ketogenic diet is not a fad diet; it's been proven to be healthy, and it supports maintainable weight loss. Rather than starving your body of calories and nutrients, you can provide it with ample energy, vitamins, and minerals while enjoying a variety of easy and delicious meals.

When you are on a standard high-carbohydrate diet, the constant assault of carbohydrates on your body causes an insulin and blood sugar response and prevents your body from burning off the digested fat and body fat. Yet when you are on a low-carbohydrate and high-fat diet, your body is burning off fat by default. Not only will it burn off the fat you consume, but it will also burn off your body fat and increase your metabolism, helping you to lose weight.

The rate of your weight loss can be customized, depending on how much of a caloric deficit you are eating. It is unhealthy to lose more than two to three pounds a week, so if after the first two weeks of the ketogenic diet you are losing more than this, then adjust your caloric deficit so that you are losing weight at a slightly slower pace. Though you may lose quite a bit the first couple of weeks in water weight, this should not concern you.

If you are already at your ideal weight or need to gain weight, you can accomplish that on the ketogenic diet as well simply by adjusting your caloric intake. Some people may consume twelve-hundred calories a day, others may consume sixteen-hundred, while others two-thousand. It all depends on the needs of your individual body, your doctor's recommendations, and whether or not you have an eating disorder.

Lower Your Cholesterol

We are used to hearing about how bad fats are for us, that they cause disease and clog our arteries. Ever since the war on fat in the 1990s and early 2000s, people have been afraid of fat, even from health sources. While there was a little truth to this, certain fats, such as trans fats, are bad for you, and there are many healthy fats as well. Yet fats such as those found in avocados, olives, sesame seeds, coconut, and nuts have been found to have amazing health benefits and weight loss promoting qualities. The ketogenic diet and these healthy sources of fats have even been shown to lower dangerous cholesterol, increase healthy cholesterol, and lower the risk of developing cardiovascular diseases.

If you have heard about the ketogenic diet raising cholesterol, it was most likely a misunderstanding, as this has never been shown to be true. On the contrary, multiple studies have shown the cholesterol-lowering properties of the ketogenic diet. The good cholesterol, which the ketogenic diet does raise, is necessary to lower bad cholesterol. This type of cholesterol boosts the absorption of vitamin D, manages hormones, and aids in the digestion of food. Good cholesterol, known as HDL, is completely harmless and promotes increased health.

There are actually two types of dangerous cholesterol, not one. These are LDL and the lesser known VLDL. These cause a buildup of plaque in the arteries and increase the risk of heart attack. On one study of the ketogenic diet, sixty-six obese patients who experienced high cholesterol went on the ketogenic diet and were able to lose weight, increase good cholesterol, lower bad cholesterol, as well as blood glucose and triglycerides. The study was deemed successful and that the ketogenic diet was shown to be a valuable treatment against high cholesterol and heart disease.

Reduce Aging

As we previously discussed, the mitochondrial cells can utilize amino acids, fatty acids, and glucose for fuel. These cells are required to produce ninety percent of the energy our body needs, and we are unable to survive without them. If these cells are not thriving, then neither can we.

While incredibly powerful and necessary, sometimes while converting fuel into energy for our cells, electrons can escape. This process will cause dangerous free radicals to form, and worse yet, these are the most dangerous type of free radicals, known as reactive oxygen species.

While this process is a natural part of aging and happens without most people being aware, it does cause cellular damage and degradation. Thankfully, the ketogenic diet can fight against this process by increasing the number of mitochondrial cells, increasing the cell's ability to convert energy efficiently, and it contains many powerful antioxidants which neutralize and remove these free radicals. This not only slows down the aging of your skin but your entire body and mind.

Treat Epilepsy and Non-Epileptic Seizures

The ketogenic diet has amazing benefits for treating seizures, both those caused by epilepsy and those that are not. In fact, the ketogenic diet was created nearly one-hundred years ago in order to treat epilepsy before anticonvulsants were created. While the ketogenic diet declined with the discovery of anticonvulsant drugs, it made a resurgence once people realized that drugs are ineffective in many people. While the ketogenic diet alone is not for everyone with uncontrolled epilepsy, it has been shown to greatly reduce seizures in many causes. This is especially great as anticonvulsants have a high rate of side effects, including drowsiness, sleepiness, and mental fatigue. These symptoms get in the way of life and even many people's jobs, making it hard to stay on the anticonvulsants, even if they are needed. Thankfully, the ketogenic diet provides people with more options.

There have been countless studies demonstrating the success of treating seizures and epilepsy with the ketogenic diet. In one study that took place at Trinity College between the years 2001 and 2006, there were one-hundred and forty-five participants. All of these participants were resistant to drug therapy in the past. Out of these patients, seven percent experienced a reduction of more than ninety percent in seizure activity. Thirty-eight percent of the people experienced an improvement of over fifty percent reduction in seizure activity.

While for most people on the ketogenic diet the body will provide ample ketones for their needs, those with neurological and neurodegenerative diseases may want to boost their ketones even more to protect their brains from potential damage caused by the illness. In this case, MCT oil (medium-chain triglycerides) and exogenous ketones have been found to provide benefits and may further reduce seizure activity. While some children who have sensitive stomachs may not be able to handle the ketogenic diet, while not as effective, MCT and exogenous ketones along may provide a small amount of benefit. This is because both of these products increase the number of ketones available to protect the brain; therefore, preventing seizures.

Reduce Your Risk of Cancer

While most of our cells can use ketones as a fuel source rather than glucose, this is not true of cancer and tumor cells. This means that when you are on the ketogenic diet, the extremely low amount of glucose in your body, as well as the production of ketones, can starve cancer and tumor cells of energy to grow. Some studies have even shown that within a few days of beginning the ketogenic diet, tumor cells, whether cancerous or not, have been shown to begin shrinking. It has also been shown to halt the growth of tumors, improving symptoms and increasing the effectiveness of chemotherapy. All of these benefits from the ketogenic diet for treating cancer have been shown to be reversed if the person discontinues the ketogenic diet.

Treat Alzheimer's Disease

Age-related diseases have dramatically increased over the years, and Alzheimer's is the most common and one of the most debilitating of these diseases. Startling, there are nearly forty-four million people worldwide who have either Alzheimer's disease or related dementia, and out of these people, Alzheimer's Disease International estimates that one in four will be diagnosed.

Not only is this disease difficult on the person diagnosed, but on the family as well. It not only takes a toll on the family's emotions, time, and finances but it in the year of 2016, 15.9 million family members provided care at an estimated 18.2 billable hours, which is 240 billion dollars.

The worst news is that Alzheimer's disease is the sixth leading cause of death in the United States, and typical life expectancy after diagnosis is only four to eight years. Startlingly, between the years of 2000 and 2014, there was an eighty-nine percent increase in deaths from Alzheimer's disease, and it is estimated that between 2017 and 2025 there will be a 14% increase in the disease.

This disease causes the neurons in the brain to develop insulin resistance, which makes it difficult for them to absorb glucose and therefore stave for fuel. Thankfully, not only do ketones act as a non-glucose fuel source for these cells, but the diet has also been shown to decrease insulin resistance. Not only will this provide the cells with ketones for fuel, but by treating the insulin resistance, they will better be able to absorb the glucose that is provided to them through the gluconeogenesis process.

One study was conducted on twenty adult participants who lived with either Alzheimer's disease or other cognitive impairment diseases. In this study, the participants were given either an MCT oil drink, which increases ketone levels, or a placebo. Within ninety minutes of drinking the MCT drink, people's ketones increased significantly, and they displayed great improvements in symptoms, whereas the placebo-control group did not improve.

In another study, a patient with Alzheimer's disease went on a treatment protocol with coconut oil and MCT oil for a twenty-month period. The patient experienced great improvement and success. They improved fourteen points on the scale of Activities of Daily Living and six points on the Alzheimer's Disease Assessment Scale-

Cognitive. The patient experienced a remarkable improvement in mood, word finding, recalling events, social participation, tremors, and gait during this time. MRI scans conducted throughout the test period displayed that his brain experienced no decline during the twenty-month treatment period.

A study that compared the effects of high-carbohydrate diets and low-carbohydrate diets on senior adults found that the participants on a low-carbohydrate diet showed improved functioning. These patients experienced a loss in fat around the abdomen as well, weight loss, as well as improved fasting insulin, memory performance, and fasting glucose. This improvement was concluded to be the result of increased ketones from the diet.

Reduce the Symptoms of Polycystic Ovary Syndrome

PCOS, otherwise known as polycystic ovary syndrome, is one of the most common endocrine disorders. This condition causes many symptoms, including hair growth, weight gain, insulin resistance, hyperinsulinemia, fatigue, irregular menstrual periods, and infertility. Yet the cause of this disorder is unknown, though chronic inflammation, increased insulin, excessive androgen, and genetics all may play an impact on the cause of this disorder. To reduce the risks associated with PCOS later on, it is important to receive early diagnosis and treatment.

Thankfully, despite much still being unknown about this condition, it has been shown that the ketogenic diet and exercise may help, as well as decreasing abdominal fat, improving insulin sensitivity, and increasing fertility.

Many people with polycystic ovary syndrome experience symptoms that affect their mental health, which can greatly impact their lives. Although, one study has found that people with PCOS who went on a low-carbohydrate and high-protein diet experienced a significant improvement in mental health symptoms. However, the people who went on a high-carbohydrate and high-protein diet did not experience any improvement.

In another study, after twenty-four weeks on the ketogenic diet, people diagnosed with PCOS experienced an average of reduced fasting insulin by fifty-four percent, twelve percent improvement in weight, thirty-six percent reduction of free testosterone, and two of the five people in the study who had previously been infertile were able to become pregnant.

Lastly, one study found that low-carbohydrate diets can improve ovulation, hormone balances, fertility, and circulating insulin in people diagnosed with PCOS.

Aids in the Management of Multiple Sclerosis

This debilitating chronic disease affects about four-hundred-thousand people in the United States alone and is three to four times more likely to affect women than men. This disease causes damage to the nerves, which then prevents communication between the body and brain. While it can affect everyone differently and at different speeds, some of the symptoms include vision loss, movement difficulties, memory impairment, numbness, reduced balance, and more.

The ketogenic diet has been proven to have many health-promoting benefits, and many of these pair perfectly against the symptoms of multiple sclerosis. For instance, it can aid in reducing inflammation, repairing cells, protecting the brain, boosting memory, and more.

One randomized and controlled study found that forty-eight people with multiple sclerosis who went on the ketogenic diet experienced a significant improvement in symptoms and disease management. These improvements were even more pronounced with the ketogenic diet was paired with intermittent fasting.

Relieve the Symptoms of Mental Illness

Mental illness is incredibly prevalent yet stigmatized greatly. Because of this, sadly, fifty-six percent of people do not seek medical care, despite over forty-million Americans living with some type of mental illness. The ableism in society leads people to perpetuate the idea that those with mental illness are violent, whereas most are not and people with mental illness are much more likely to experience violence rather than perpetrating it. Many mental illnesses can get in the way of every aspect of life, both in someone's personal and professional life. Mental illness does not take a break.

While many more studies still need to be done, it has been shown that the ketogenic diet may benefit people living with a number of mental illnesses or symptoms.

In a study on depression in rats, it was found that the ketogenic diet was equally as effective as antidepressants. The rats in the study no longer exhibited the behavior of despair, and they became more mobile. Another similar study found that it was able to help stabilize the mood. Yet take this with a grain of salt as it is not a human trial, and even if it was, you should never go off of antidepressants without a doctor's care.

Bipolar disorder affects over five and a half million Americans, and yet being one of the more prevalent mental disorders, it is still greatly misunderstood and stigmatized. Although one study has found that two women diagnosed with type II bipolar disorder were able to experience an improvement in mood stabilization on the ketogenic diet, that was more effective than what they were able to achieve with medication. This was also a long-term study, where one woman was studied on the diet for two years and the other for three years.

While autism is not a mental illness, it can cause mood disorders and anxiety disorders. Studies showing the management of mood and anxiety for autistic people with the ketogenic diet are limited; however, some have shown that it may help and decrease social stress.

As you can see, there are many reasons in which to choose the ketogenic diet. Study after study has found it to be a safe option for most people while also being effective in improving overall health.

Whether your goal is to protect your mental health, lower your cholesterol, reduce your risk of cancer, or lose weight, the ketogenic diet can help.

Chapter 3: The Ketosis Process

Restricting carbohydrates in order to reach a state of ketosis and the many benefits ketones provide is the founding principle of the ketogenic diet. While this diet is simple and easy, for people new to it, there may be confusion on what ketosis actually is, how to know if you are in ketosis, and any side effects it might have. In this chapter, we will go in-depth on ketosis and what you can expect.

What Ketosis Is

While many people are unaware of the ketosis process, it is a natural metabolic state in which the body will create ketones for fuel, due to a lack of glucose. While this state can be entered into by fasting, the most popular, easy, and maintainable method for ketosis is through restricting carbohydrate intake on the ketogenic diet. With this method, you still receive all of the nutrients your body requires. It takes some people longer than others to enter into a state of sustained ketosis, depending on their food intake, activity levels, and health. For instance, people with diabetes take longer to enter a ketosis state. Yet you can expect to be in truly sustained ketosis within a day or up to a week and a half. This state is defined by having a blood ketone level of 0.5 mmol/L.

This state of ketosis has many benefits, aside from protecting against disease and aiding in weight loss, including decreasing hunger, sustaining energy, and improving cognitive function.

You might be wondering why the time it takes to go into sustained ketosis may vary. This is because it depends on how much glycogen, which is the form of glucose which is stored in your muscles and liver, is currently in your body and how quickly you burn through it. People on a high carbohydrate diet and eat a lot of sugary foods will have more glucose in their system than someone on a low-sugar whole food diet. Exercise will burn off this glucose quicker, so if you are an athlete, you will most likely enter ketosis quicker than most people.

While diabetics and insulin resistance may take longer to get into deep ketosis, the good news is that the ketogenic diet has been proven time and time again to treat insulin resistance. Therefore, the longer you are on it, the more your insulin and blood sugar response will improve.

The Keto Flu

For the first one to two weeks of the ketogenic diet, you can expect to go into a 'keto flu'. For some people, this is very mild, and they hardly notice the change – aside from needing to eat more frequently. Although, for many people, this truly does feel like the flu. It may be unpleasant while your body adjusts to altering to using ketones for fuel rather than glucose, but soon you will begin to notice the flu-like symptoms fade away and be replaced by higher levels of energy, decreased hunger, and other daily improvements.

Thankfully, while the symptoms of the keto flu may be bothersome, they are safe and pass quickly.

Bad Breath

We all dread bad breath, but you may have to live with it for a day or two of the ketogenic diet. This is because your body begins to produce ketones, and one of these ketones is acetone. Yet our cells are unable to utilize acetone, so instead, it is excreted through both the breath and urine. This 'keto breath' may be rather pungent, smelling similarly to nail polish remover or overripe fruit. It is not pleasant.

Thankfully, it does not last long. Your body will quickly become acclimated to creating ketones and will produce the more productive ketones beta-hydroxybutyrate and acetoacetate instead, and once it does, you will be in ketosis.

There is not much you can do about the bad breath. Just try to keep your distance from people and a lot of mints on hand for a couple of days.

Dry Mouth and Extreme Thirst

Due to restricting carbohydrates, your body will dump water weight and electrolytes rapidly. This will often cause dehydration, dry mouth, and thirst. While this is a good sign that the ketogenic diet is working for you, be sure to replenish on fluids and electrolytes. You don't want to allow the dehydration to get out of hand.

It is most commonly recommended to drink half of your body's weight in ounces. Therefore, if you weight one-hundred and fifty pounds, you will want to drink a minimum of seventy-five ounces of water a day. Although, more water than this would be ideal to ensure that you are getting enough while your body is dumping much of its stored water.

Just be sure to never drink more than a liter in the time span of an hour, as your liver is unable to process more and it would put a strain on your organs. Also, be careful to get the important electrolytes (sodium, magnesium, potassium, and calcium) along with the water, as the electrolyte molecules bind to the water molecules. This means that when water is dumped from your body, so are the electrolytes, and they need to be restored.

Increased Urination

Ketones and low levels of carbohydrate intake are both natural diuretics. Not only that but as insulin levels decrease, more water and sodium are released from the body, meaning frequent bathroom trips. This is a good sign and should even out the longer you are on the ketogenic diet.

Digestive Upset

The ketogenic diet is quite a change for people, and while a relatively simple and easy to manage change, your digestive tract may require some time to adjust. In fact, the most common side effect of the ketogenic diet is digestive upset, but with a little time or tinkering of your diet, the symptoms should go away.

Some people become badly constipated, but with a bit of tinkering, this is one easy to manage side effect. The causes are simple to fix and are usually due to dehydration, electrolyte deficiencies, or too little fiber. Thankfully, if you increase these in your diet, constipation should go away. You can find sugar-free and artificial sweetener-free electrolyte drink powders, such as Ultima Replenisher, which is an awesome option for replenishing these important minerals.

Many people may completely avoid vegetables on the ketogenic diet because they are trying to keep the net carbohydrate count low, and instead eat other things, such as nuts and dairy. While nuts and dairy have their place in a ketogenic diet, it is important to eat vegetables for their nutrition and fiber content. Stick to low-carbohydrate vegetables, such as cauliflower, broccoli, and Brussels sprouts.

You may develop diarrhea due to your body dumping excess fluids. There is not much you can do about this, but it should go away on its own shortly. Simply stay hydrated and take those electrolytes. You may also consider holding off on MCT oil products until after the diarrhea goes away, as it is more quickly digested than other sources of fat, meaning it could potentially cause diarrhea in large amounts.

While a digestive upset is one of the more common side effects of the ketogenic diet during the keto flu, don't worry – you may not even experience it. While it is common, many people still do not have either. In fact, the ketogenic diet may help people who live with chronic constipation.

Change in Hunger

During the first couple of weeks on the ketogenic diet, you may find yourself more frequently hungry, despite the food being more calorie dense. Therefore, even if your goal is to ultimately lose weight, you may want to begin with a weight-maintaining calorie count, so that way you are less likely to become hungry and stressed. That would only be a recipe for overeating later.

Thankfully, the ketogenic diet naturally suppresses hunger, which aids in weight loss. This is because while carbohydrates burn off quickly, leaving you hungry and needing to refuel, the fats on the ketogenic diet are slow burning and satisfying. By the end of the first month you should notice your hunger decreasing, and in the following months, it may even decrease further. This is especially helpful since fats are high in calories, and without this hunger reduction, it would be easy to overeat by hundreds of calories.

You will find yourself needing to eat less, feeling more energized, and able to go longer periods between meals. This is especially helpful for people living a busy life.

Increased Fatigue

Prior to beginning the sustained ketosis phase, which provides increased energy, the keto flu may cause you to experience increased fatigue, both in mind and body. Thankfully, this does not last for long and can be reduced by a few simple methods. To decrease the fatigue, try to consume ample water and electrolytes, eat as needed – be sure you are eating adequate protein – and consider light to mild exercises, such as walking or stretching, and getting plenty of sleep.

Insomnia

Difficulty falling asleep or staying asleep, otherwise known as insomnia, is something that plagues the nighttime for many people worldwide. Yet if you are someone who suddenly develops insomnia on the ketogenic diet, then it is most likely not chronic insomnia and should go away along with the keto flu.

The reason for this is because when you reduce your carbohydrate intake, your body is struggling to adapt to the new sources of fuel; therefore, it releases stress hormones on the biochemical level. While there is little you can do for that, you may try milk sleep aids as well as limiting stimulants and lowering stress. Deep breathing, yoga, meditation, and mild exercise may all help decrease your overall lifestyle stress, helping reduce a little of the stress on your body from the biochemical reaction.

This should go away as soon as you become keto-adapted, otherwise known as being in sustained ketosis, and your body can properly utilize ketones for fuel.

Tracking Ketone Levels

While not necessary, some people prefer to track their ketone levels. It can ease the mind of the person, letting them know where they are at on the scale of no ketosis to being in sustained ketosis. However, it is not recommended that you worry about your ketone levels too much because as long as you are following your macro ratio, you shouldn't have any problems entering or maintaining ketosis.

If you do decide to test for ketones, it is best to start one to two days after beginning the diet because sooner than that will not reveal anything. It is also important to remember that it will take two to three weeks to enter sustained ketosis.

One last caution: the urine sticks and breath meters, while helpful, are not completely accurate. These tests simply test the number of ketones that are being expelled from the body, not the actual number of ketones you have. Blood ketone tests are most accurate because after you have been in sustained ketosis for a while, your body will learn to produce less of an excess of ketones. Since your body learns what it needs, it will then be able to produce that, and very little more, so you will find that the numbers on urine and breath sticks go down.

Many people will panic upon seeing their ketone levels go down after being on the ketogenic diet for a couple of months, but it is in fact because they are doing so well, not because they are doing badly.

Overview of What to Expect

The process of ketosis differs from person to person, yet there is a general idea of what you may expect. Knowing what may happen can help you plan, ease your worries, and better handle what may come your way.

You shouldn't notice any changes the first day or two. If you do, it will likely only be increased hunger. To counteract this, try to include a couple of snacks to keep your energy levels up and prevent overeating on a meal later in the day.

During days three to seven, you are likely to begin noticing increased fatigue and other symptoms of the keto flu. The severity of these symptoms varies, but for some people, they are quite mild.

By the end of the first week, or during the second week, you should begin to dump excess acetone ketones and excrete them in your urine and breath. This can be tested with either breath or urine testers. If you decide to test, the urine strips are less expensive, but the breath test is more accurate.

After the second week, the bad breath should go away, your symptoms should begin to dissipate, and you should enter sustained ketosis.

By the third and fourth week, you should notice your energy levels going up, hunger decreasing, and other improvements, depending on what your individual health is like. For instance, if you have high cholesterol or insulin resistance, they will most likely begin to improve at this point.

The process of entering ketosis is different for everyone, but it doesn't have to be difficult or scary. You've got this, and you can succeed in reaching better health and a better life.

Chapter 4: Amazing Ketogenic Tips and Tricks

The ketogenic diet is not difficult. It is an easy way of life, even for people who are constantly on the run, have little income, are unable to cook, or have disabilities which impede mobility. In this chapter, we will introduce you to some simple tips and tricks to help make the ketogenic diet even simpler. With this advice, you will be on the road to success in no time.

Limit Carbohydrates

When you enter the ketogenic diet, a large part of what impacts how quickly you enter ketosis is how much glycogen you have stored in your liver and muscles. Glycogen, which is a stored version of glucose, can be kept up to two-thousand calories worth within these parts of the body. Depending on how much glycogen you have stored from your pre-ketogenic diet, how active you are, and how low you are eating carbohydrates on the ketogenic diet will affect how quickly you enter ketosis.

If you are hoping to enter ketosis as soon as possible, and therefore get over the keto flu quicker, then the best way is to limit your carbohydrate intake on the ketogenic diet as much as possible. While twenty-five net carbohydrates are the standard recommended daily amount on the ketogenic diet, you could limit it to ten or fifteen net carbohydrates to help your glycogen stores deplete faster.

Live Actively

When you first begin the ketogenic diet, and your body is attempting to adapt from being fueled off of carbohydrates and switching to using fat and ketones instead, your athletic ability and endurance may decrease slightly. Thankfully, this only lasts an average of three to four weeks, and then you can expect your exercise performance to improve. In fact, studies have shown that ketosis can actually improve your athletic ability, especially when it comes to aerobic and endurance activities.

While you may not be able to exercise to your usual degree for the first couple of weeks, exercise can help deplete your glycogen stores; therefore, increasing ketone production and aiding in pushing you into a state of ketosis sooner rather than later.

In fact, multiple studies have shown that not only does working out while in a fasted state increase ketone levels but if you exercise while on the ketogenic diet, the rate that ketones are produced is increased as well. One study found that when on the ketogenic diet, if you exercise prior to a meal rather than afterward, the blood ketone levels can be one-hundred and thirty-seven percent to three-hundred and fourteen percent higher.

Include Coconut or MCT Oil

Not only does coconut oil provide you with many health benefits, but it contains many medium-chain triglycerides, also known as MCT oil. Consuming either coconut oil, or pure MCT oil, can help increase ketone levels, energy, and satiety.

Unlike most other fats, medium-chain triglycerides can be rapidly digested and then delivered to the liver where they are used as fuel or transmuted into ketones. While you can buy pure MCT oil, coconut oil contains about fifty percent of medium-chain triglycerides, making it a wonderful health-promoting and energizing option. The remaining portion of coconut oil is lauric acid, which has also been shown in studies to produce a sustained level of ketones; therefore, the coconut oil is a combination of two powerful fats for ketosis.

Coconut oil has also been shown in a wide range of studies to improve the symptoms of Alzheimer's disease, protect the nervous system, reduce the frequency of seizures in people with epilepsy, and increase weight loss.

If you plan on adding coconut or MCT oil to your diet, it is a good plan to introduce them slowly so that your body can adjust. If you add these fats too quickly, your digestive system will not be able to easily digest them, inducing possible diarrhea or stomach cramps. Thankfully, if you slowly start adding one teaspoon of coconut oil before eventually working up to two or three tablespoons over the course of a week or two, you shouldn't experience any digestive upset.

Prioritize Sleep

If you are sleep deprived or oversleeping, your body will increase the production of stress hormones. Not only can this affect your overall stress level, but it can prevent you from losing weight and sometimes even cause weight gain. Therefore, it is important to ensure that you are sleeping the recommended number of hours. Studies have shown that less than seven hours or more than nine hours will increase these stress hormones; therefore, it is best to find what suits your needs within that time span.

If you find you have difficulty falling or staying asleep, there are some common recommendations which help many people, though you may need to play around with it until you find the solution which helps you. The American Sleep Association recommends a number of tips in order to improve sleep hygiene. Some of these tips and tricks include:

• Wake up and go to sleep at the same time daily. If you have difficulty falling asleep, many sleep specialists will recommend starting by only focusing on waking up at the same time daily, then falling asleep should eventually fall into place. Ideally, this schedule should stay the same on most days. Try not to alter it by more than twenty minutes, if possible.

• Try to avoid naps. Each person only needs a certain amount of sleep, and if you nap, then you will need less sleep when nighttime comes. If you absolutely must nap, try to limit them to only thirty minutes.

• Don't lay in bed unable to sleep. If you find yourself with your mind racing and unable to sleep for twenty minutes, then get out of bed and do something else, such as reading a book. Lying in bed will only further the insomnia cycle. Yet if you are out of bed and doing something relaxing, your body will learn to settle down when you get back into bed. It is important, though, that when you get out of bed when having insomnia, you avoid the TV and computer, as the blue light emitted by these have been shown to trigger insomnia.

• Don't chill in bed. It has been shown that people who spend more time in bed watching TV, reading, writing, or whatever, have increased insomnia. If you can, it is much better to do these things in a chair or on the couch and reserve your bed for sleeping.

• Be careful of stimulants and other items which may affect your sleep, such as caffeine, cigarettes, alcohol, and medications.

• Regular sleep can help improve sleep quality, but it is important to avoid strenuous exercise within four hours of bedtime for most people. There may be the occasional person who sleeps better by first working out, but for the general population, this will only promote difficulty sleeping. This is because strenuous exercise increases endorphins, which energizes the body and makes falling asleep more difficult.

• Keep your bedroom a quiet and comfortable space. Lights, even the slight light emitted from a cell phone or car lights, will disturb your sleep cycle. Therefore, try to keep the room as dark as possible by utilizing room darkening curtains and keeping all lights off. People are also shown to sleep better in a cool room, so if possible keep the thermostat low during the evening.

Cook Large Batches of Food

While cooking can be greatly limited on the ketogenic diet with the addition of precooked meats and microwave-steamed vegetables, that doesn't mean you won't ever need to cook. Although, if you are limited on time or energy, cooking in large batches can save you energy, time, and money. Simply cook more food than you need and store it in the fridge or freezer. If you desire, you can simply cook two or three servings at a time to store in the fridge, or you can make enough food to last you two or three weeks and store it in the freezer. This is wonderful for people on the go, as you simply have to remove it from the freezer and thaw it out in the microwave.

Get Your Carbohydrates from Vegetables

While you can get some of your daily net carbohydrates from dairy, nuts, or other items, you should try to keep most of your carbohydrates coming from low-starch vegetables and low-sugar fruits. Cabbage, kale, broccoli, avocado, olives, strawberries, blackberries – there are some wonderful fruit and vegetable options on the ketogenic diet, and it is important to not forsake these in order to eat "low-carb" packaged foods, such as low-carbohydrate tortillas. You need nutrition and fiber that comes from these amazing fruits and vegetables.

Invest in a Kitchen Scale

Accurately tracking your food intake for your macro ratio is incredibly important on the ketogenic diet, especially during the beginning phase. Many people may just eyeball what they think is the correct proportion, but it is inaccurate and results in them being kicked out of ketosis. People will be frustrated by not understanding why their weight has stalled, only to learn it is because they were not weighing and tracking their food. For instance, if you eyeball what you think is the correct amount of almond butter, you could accidentally consume an extra two tablespoons over the course of a day. While two tablespoons may not seem like much, it contains two hundred calories and six net carbohydrates.

A kitchen scale is the most accurate way in which to track how much food you are consuming, and they are simple to use. Thankfully, these scales are rather inexpensive, and you can get an inexpensive one between ten and twenty-five dollars.

Take Exogenous Ketones

Like coconut and MCT oil, exogenous ketones can help you increase the number of ketone bodies you have and make the process of going into ketosis more easy and quick. In fact, including some exogenous ketones in your diet can greatly improve your ketogenic journey by giving you more energy and helping your body adapt to the process of ketosis sooner than it otherwise would.

The best type of exogenous ketones and the most common on the market is beta-hydroxybutyrate, otherwise known as BHB. These are the most effective form of ketones which your body can easily use as fuel and energy.

While many people dread the idea of the keto flu, especially if they are busy with work or family, the addition of exogenous ketones has helped many people avoid this phenomenon. They may be a little pricey, but if you can afford it, then it could be worth adding exogenous ketones to your diet for at least the first two weeks of the ketogenic diet.

Keep Snacks on Hand

The last thing you want is to be tired and hungry, just needing a snack but with nothing to eat. Therefore, to help you stick to your diet and prevent overeating in the evenings, it is best to keep snacks on hand. Some great snacks are cheese, boiled eggs, sandwich meat, beef jerky, nuts, fat bombs, previously prepared guacamole, or precooked bacon.

Eating out on the Ketogenic Diet

For some people eating out is a regular occurrence or at least something they enjoy doing with loved ones or coworkers from time to time. Thankfully, just because you are on a diet doesn't mean you have to give up on eating out. Salads without croutons are often wonderful choices, but there are many other options as well.

Steak, fish, and shellfish are all low-carbohydrate options as long as they are not breaded. You can also often have them with a side of a low-starch vegetable.

If you are at a sushi restaurant, rather than ordering sushi which contains rice, order sashimi. Sashimi is simply the raw fish, which you can then dip in soy sauce or wasabi. Don't worry; it's not bland! Eating the sashimi in this way allows you to appreciate the flavors and freshness fully, and it is quite popular in Japan.

If you feel like a burger, most places will accommodate you by giving you one with lettuce rather than a bun. Eating a burger either over a salad or wrapped in lettuce in this way is incredibly satisfying and equally tasty.

Breakfast options may be more limited, but you can always enjoy eggs, cheese, bacon, and breakfast sausage!

Chapter 5: Pairing the Ketogenic Diet with Exercise

Most people are taught that in order to lose weight, they need to restrict calories and wear themselves out with an excessive amount of strenuous exercise. While this may seem effective, after all, you are consuming fewer calories than you are expanding, it often produced fewer results than people expect. The scale barely moves, you feel hungry, and you are worn out.

You may think that increasing the amount of exercise will help you shed more pounds, but rather, it will cause you to be hungrier, resulting in overeating. It will also increase the strain on our cells and the amount of inflammation in our bodies.

While this method of weight loss causes stress on both the mind and body, it does not have to be this way on the ketogenic diet. Unlike most diets, you will find that you feel fuller longer, require less food, and have energy. This will not only help you work out better, but it will help prevent you from overeating and undoing your hard work.

As if that wasn't enough, scientific studies have shown that exercise is incredibly more effective on the ketogenic diet. This is great news for people with limited time, energy, or desire to exercise. In one study, it was found that people who exercise on the ketogenic diet burn two to three times more fat during exercise than people on a high-carbohydrate diet. This is because the process of ketosis will help your body burn off body fat rather than glycogen in the muscles.

The ketogenic diet will also provide you increased and sustained energy during your workouts. While most people will have their blood sugar drop, due to burning off glucose and glycogen, because you are using ketones and fat as a fuel source, you will find that your blood sugar stays stable, keeping your energy up. This is especially helpful for people who use endurance exercises.

However, while there are many benefits to working out on the ketogenic diet, and study after study has shown it to be more effective and maintainable than people working out on standard diets, slowly work yourself into it while you adjust. If you begin both your ketogenic diet and a new exercise regimen simultaneously, you are more likely to find yourself worn out, especially during the keto flu period.

Thankfully, by the end of the first or second week, you should notice your energy levels going up, and by the end of the first month, you should be back to full active abilities. It is best during this first month of the ketogenic diet to stick to light and moderate exercise rather than strenuous. Although, if bodybuilding or HIIT training is important to you, you can make these easier in the first month if you incorporate exogenous ketones into your diet. As mentioned earlier, these will help your body adjust to ketosis quicker and prevent the keto flu, aiding in getting you on your feet for the first month of the ketogenic diet.

While the type of exercise you can do on the ketogenic diet is not limited, some are not ideal with the standard ketogenic diet. For instance, the targeted or cyclical ketogenic diets are best suited if you are into bodybuilding or HIIT training, rather than the standard ketogenic diet.

This is because short and high-intensity workouts, which take between ten seconds and two minutes, rely upon the glucose in our muscles. You may be able to get by without eating many carbohydrates, but you will find your stamina and strength more limited. Thankfully, with the cyclical and targeted ketogenic diets, you can still reap the many benefits of the diet, but with enough carbohydrates to fuel your workout.

If you are someone who uses aerobic exercises or anything that is less than strenuous, then you should have all of the stamina and power you need with the standard ketogenic diet, as these types of exercises do not require glucose and can be fueled completely with ketones, fat, and protein.

Stretching and Flexibility Exercises

There are many benefits to flexibility exercises such as yoga, Pilates, and tai chi. Not only are these calming and helpful for your mental health, but they strengthen and lengthen muscles, helping to increase your range of motion and decrease the risk of injury. This is especially important as we age and are more likely to develop debilitating injuries. However, it can also be helpful for people who enjoy moderate or strenuous exercises to incorporate some flexibility exercises as well. It will promote their performance and lessen the risk of them developing a workout-related injury.

It is important to remember that while these flexibility exercises appear simple, many of them have more to them than meets the eye. You are unable to appreciate how much control and strength they require until you try them. Therefore, it is important to not jump into difficult stretches or routines too quickly; otherwise, you will cause an injury. Begin with beginner level routines, and gradually work your way up. If you are unsure how to approach this on your own, there are a wide variety of classes available at gyms and yoga studios.

You have most likely heard your entire life that you should stretch before you exercise, but it has actually been found that this is ineffective. Rather than using these stretching and flexibility exercises before a strenuous workout, it is better to use them afterward to help your body cool down at a steady pace. Instead, before you use a strenuous workout, it is best to warm up with some mild jogging or something else that requires the muscles you will be using. For instance, if you play football, you can warm up by jogging around the field and passing the ball back and forth to teammates for five to ten minutes until your muscles are warmed up and supple.

While flexibility exercises and stretching have many health benefits, some of the most common include stress relief, improved sleep, decreased muscle strain, increased muscle control, improved muscle strength and tone, decreased muscle tension, improved posture, decreased joint strain, improved lung function, and reduced inflammation.

Aerobics and Cardio

Aerobics and cardio are a wonderful option, not only because they can be attained while on the standard ketogenic diet without any carbohydrates required, but because they have a wonderful ability to strengthen our bodies and increase our health. Some of these health benefits include, but are not limited to, strengthening muscles, improving lung function, increasing endorphins, promoting better sleep quality, raising dopamine, managing arthritis pain, increasing joint range of motion, raising serotonin, improving skin health, increasing blood flow to the brain, raising norepinephrine, improving memory, controlling blood sugar, improving body composition, and, of course, increasing weight loss.

Some examples of aerobic cardio exercises include jogging, cycling, swimming, running, boxing, power walking, dancing, hiking, rowing, stair stepping, and recreational sports.

When you are doing these exercises, it is important to keep your heart rate in a targeted zone, depending on your age. This zone is different for everyone and is recommended to be fifty to seventy percent of two-hundred and twenty minus your age. This means that if you are thirty, then it would be one-hundred and ninety, making your individual target zone between nighty-five and one-hundred and thirty-three. Exercise watches are incredibly helpful to make sure you keep your heart rate in the correct zone, and there are some pretty decent inexpensive options on the market if you don't get one with all the bells and whistles.

When you are new to cardio, it is best to start out at your minimum heart rate zone for ten to fifteen minutes, and slowly increase the intensity and length of time as you adapt. You can push yourself by slowly increasing both the heart rate and time span in five-minute increments a week. Eventually, it is ideal to work up to thirty minutes to forty-five minutes, but if you are only able to exercise for twenty minutes, that is okay. Remember: exercise is more effective for weight loss on the ketogenic diet.

High-Intensity Interval Training (HIIT)

While aerobics and cardio have the most health benefits when completed for over thirty minutes, HIIT training is unique because it is an incredibly high-intensity all-out exercise that can be completed in twenty minutes. While it may not take as long as cardio to complete a HIIT can spend less time working out while getting even more of a boost to your weight loss goal and health. This is especially helpful in the busy lives we live in this day and age, and for people who simply hate exercise and want to get it over as quickly as possible.

If you are interested in attempting high-intensity interval training, then it is best paired with the targeted ketogenic diet since it is most effective when you have a bit of glycogen in your system, but it doesn't require enough to need the cyclical ketogenic diet.

In one study, it was found that people who performed HIIT routines three times weekly for twenty minutes each were able to lose an average of 4.4 pounds of body fat during a twelve-week period, and this is without any dietary changes. This alone is wonderful news, as exercise without diet often yields few results in weight loss. But, it is even better because seventeen percent of the fat lost was the most dangerous type of fat, visceral fat, which surrounds the organs and causes disease.

Another study was conducted to compare the difference of lung control and oxygen usage in both HIIT and cardio routines on stationary bikes. On average, people's lungs and oxygen improved by twenty-five percent, but while the cardio group was required to exercise for two hours a week to attain this, the HIIT group only needed to exercise half of that time to reach the same benefits.

A study on the number of calories burned during exercise compared HIIT to weight training, biking and running. The study revealed that those who used HIIT as opposed to the other forms of exercise were able to burn an average of twenty-five to thirty percent more calories.

Some of the other benefits of HIIT exercise is improved blood pressure, reduced blood sugar, improved insulin resistance, increased muscle strength, reduced heart rate, increased endurance, boosted metabolism, and it even continues to burn calories even after you stop working out.

But, what does a HIIT workout look like? There are many ways in which you can customize a HIIT routine, but one simple example is if you warm up by walking for five minutes, and then sprinting as fast as you possibly can for thirty full seconds. You can then cool down with a four-minute walk before repeating the process a few times.

Bodybuilding

If you worry about your ability to pack on muscle and body build on the ketogenic diet, there is no need to fear. Bodybuilding can be accomplished on the ketogenic diet, both with the targeted ketogenic diet and the cyclical ketogenic diet. If you are a beginner, it is highly recommended to begin with the targeted ketogenic diet rather than cyclical; otherwise, you are unlikely to burn off all of the glucose and glycogen in your system, kicking you out of ketosis. Although, if you are an advanced bodybuilder who works out three or more times a week, then the cyclical ketogenic diet is right up your alley.

If you would like, you can even increase your protein level on any of the ketogenic diets in order to boost your bodybuilding. To eat a high-protein version of the diets, simply consume between one and 1.3 grams of protein for each pound of body weight, but be sure to include the calories from this protein into your daily macro ratio and calorie count. Some good sources of protein for this include beef, chicken, turkey, lamb, fatty fish, shrimp, sardines, eggs, nuts, whole-fat dairy, and tofu.

Chapter 6: The Ketogenic Diet and Intermittent Fasting

Some people will go on fad fasting cleanses, that last one to two weeks. These are incredibly unhealthy, as they deprive the body of important nutrients. However, intermittent fasting is done for much shorter periods of time and is simply lengthening the time between meals. Many people only fast for eight to twelve hours with intermittent fasting. If you are still unsure about intermittent fasting, there are many studies not only showing it to be a healthy approach to weight loss but that it can also greatly boost your health.

Intermittent fasting and the ketogenic diet work wonderfully as a pair, even better than they do on their own. This is because not only do they boost the health benefits of each other, but the ketogenic diet also makes intermittent fasting easier by keeping you sustained, full, and energized while you fast. Rather than struggling to fast, it feels natural and simple.

Some people will even begin their ketogenic journey by starting with a fast so that they can more quickly burn off the glycogen and enter ketosis. While this is a great option for people who want to enter ketosis as rapidly as possible, it is also much more difficult to fast until you are in a state of sustained ketosis. In fact, it is commonly not recommended to attempt fasting until you have been on the ketogenic diet for a month. However, if you want to enter ketosis as soon as possible without the use of exogenous ketones, it is an available option.

Many health benefits of intermittent fasting have been briefly mentioned, but what *are* some of these? The sheer power of intermittent fasting is amazing, some of the health benefits include, but are not limited to, the following:

Weight Loss

When you are in a fed state, your body will naturally burn off the calories you have just eaten. But when you are in a fasted state, your body can utilize the stored fat, otherwise known as adipose and body fat, for fuel and energy. Between the restriction of calories during a fast and the ability to burn off body fat, it has been found to be a wonderful tool for weight loss.

In one study, various participants practiced intermittent fasting for three to twenty-four weeks during 2014. This study showed that each participant decreased their body weight by an average of three to eight percent.

Slow Down Aging

When fasting, the number of ketones and mitochondrial cells are increased. This increase can help your cells function and heal better, decreasing aging. While more studies are required, this has been proven to be true in studies both on animals and humans.

Increased Growth Hormone

While most people, unless they have an endocrine disorder, do not consider their hormones, they play a vital role in every aspect of our lives. One of these incredibly important hormones is the human growth hormone, which is produced in the pituitary gland. The hormone is responsible for regulating the health of the tissues in our brain, bone density, muscle mass, cell growth, and cell regeneration.

This hormone increases up to five times its standard levels when we are fasting, which can ease the burden of aging, improve the health of our cells, aid in weight loss, increase healing, improve cardiovascular health, and much more. This is one of the most powerful effects of intermittent fasting and can't be over-appreciated.

Reduce Inflammation

Inflammation is an important part of the immune system. Without it, our cells would be vulnerable to attack from foreign invaders and unable to fight off illness. Although, increased levels of chronic inflammation are equally as dangerous as a lack of inflammation. This is because chronically high levels of inflammation have been shown to cause and worsen many diseases.

Thankfully, not only does the ketogenic diet balance inflammation levels but as does intermittent fasting. Studies have even shown it to improve rheumatoid arthritis, heart disease, and cancer.

In one study, it was found that people who practice intermittent fasting have inflammation lowered to a significant degree, which could be helpful not only in chronically ill individuals but also in healthy people who are trying to improve their health as they age and prevent illness.

Treat Insulin Resistance

Insulin resistance is known to cause weight gain, raise blood pressure, increase blood triglycerides, and often goes hand in hand with or leads to diabetes. Thankfully, studies have found that both the ketogenic diet and intermittent fasting are effective in treating and reducing insulin resistance. Treating insulin resistance can help decrease blood sugar spikes and crashes, help your body more effectively transport glucose, lessen your risk of developing diabetes, and improve diabetes.

Reduces Muscle Loss

When people diet by restricting their caloric intake, they often lose lean muscle mass. Luckily, weight loss does not have to mean losing your important muscle mass. A study conducted in 2011 found that while both caloric restriction and intermittent fasting lead to similar amounts of fat loss, intermittent fasting caused less of a loss in muscle mass than caloric restrictions.

Increase Brain Function

The research of intermittent fasting on the human brain is limited, but animal studies show us that it could have a profound effect on brain health. Intermittent fasting has been linked to improvements in both Alzheimer's disease and Parkinson's disease, as well as other neurodegenerative illnesses.
A study on intermittent fasting and its effects on mice found that after eleven months, they experienced not only an improvement in brain function but even an improvement in the very structure of the brain. In another study, it was found that intermittent fasting can improve nerve cell growth, cognitive function, and overall neurological health.

Improve Heart Health

Heart disease is one of the most common causes of death and affects people around the world. In fact, heart disease is so severe that it causes 31.5 percent of deaths across the world. Thankfully, while this is an incredibly prevalent problem, diet, exercise, and other lifestyle changes have been shown greatly to reduce your risk and improve your heart health. One of the lifestyle changes that has been shown to improve your heart health is intermittent fasting.

A study conducted on an alternate day fasting for a period of eight weeks showed great results on heart health. In fact, LDL cholesterol was lowered by twenty-five percent, and blood triglycerides were reduced by thirty-two percent.

In an additional study, it was found that over one hundred adults who were categorized as "obese" were significantly able to reduce their cholesterol, blood pressure, and blood triglycerides in only three weeks.

Reduce Seizure Activity

The connection of fasting to help control seizures has been shown in studies for over a hundred years. In fact, this connection is what led researchers to develop the ketogenic diet. Pairing both the ketogenic diet and intermittent fasting is powerful for people with epilepsy, as the ketogenic diet naturally causes ketone production, and then intermittent fasting increases this ketone production. A large number of ketones protect the brain, which then reduces or prevents seizure activity.

Boost Energy Levels

Intermittent fasting increases the production of mitochondrial cells, which then produce fuel for your body and increase energy levels. This is especially important as mitochondrial cells provide ninety percent of the energy our body requires. This not only increases your physical and mental energy levels while fasting but afterward as well.

Increase Brain Cells

Intermittent fasting has been shown to increase neurogenesis in the brain. Scientific studies have shown that this process causes the growth of vital brain cells and nerve tissue. This is helpful as it boosts mood, increases memory, improves focus ability, and increases brain performance. If you find you are someone who is constantly struggling to focus or struggling with mental health, then this will especially help you. This can happen thanks to the brain-derived neurotrophic factor, or BDNF, which stimulates cell growth in the cortex, hippocampus, basal forebrain, and the nervous system.

Reduce the Risk of and Treat Cancer

While more studies need to be done, as they are still in the animal trial stage, the effects of intermittent fasting on cancer are promising. This is logical, as the ketogenic diet has also been proven to treat and prevent cancer and they both have similar health-promoting effects. Intermittent fasting has also been shown to remove free radicals, which have been tied to the formation of cancer cells.

Studies conducted on rats have shown that fasting every other day may help cease the production of tumors, prevent cancer, and increase the effective power of chemotherapy.

As you can see, there are many benefits to practicing intermittent fasting, but how do you actually accomplish it in a healthy and easy way? Don't worry; let's walk you through step by step.

Intermittent Fasting Fundamentals

Understanding how intermittent fasting can have these many health benefits and how to utilize it requires an understanding of the fundamentals.

The first part to understand is the difference between the fed state and the fasted state. The fed state begins after you eat a meal and will last an average of five hours until your body has fully digested the meal. During this state, your body will burn off the calories you have just eaten and is unlikely to burn off the stored adipose tissue.

Three to five hours after you have eaten, you will go into a post-absorptive state. During this phase, your insulin levels will be lower, and you can more easily burn adipose tissue.

The fasted state does not begin for twelve hours after eating, which most people do not achieve on the standard Western diet. This increases fat loss without much effort, even if you are consuming the same number of calories in a day as you otherwise would.

Some people may worry that fasting is supposedly the same as starvation, but this is untrue. Short-term fasting is completely safe when you are eating a healthy and balanced diet, such as the ketogenic diet. Think about this: there is nothing unhealthy about going without eating between dinner and breakfast, and it is the same with intermittent fasting. As long as you are careful to eat enough calories and nutrients, intermittent fasting has been proven to be healthy.

There are different types of fasts, and you can use whichever one is best suited to your lifestyle and preference. However, it is important to remember that if you are struggling with hunger, don't force yourself. If you force yourself to fast, then you are likely to overeat later on. Instead, fasting should be a natural and easy process. Eat when you are hungry and fast when you are not, it is that simple.

Skip a Meal

The most simple and easy method of intermittent fasting is skipping a meal. To accomplish this type of fasting, simply skip a meal whenever you aren't hungry. With this method, you shouldn't feel hungry or tired, and you don't have to worry about fitting it into a schedule.

This method is especially beneficial for beginners, who are not yet ready or confident enough to try a longer fast or a scheduled fast. If you slowly work in skipping meals, then you will find scheduled fasts easier later on.

Twelve-Hour Fast

The twelve-hour window fast often referred to as the twelve/twelve fast, is one of the easiest methods of scheduled fast. The fasting window isn't as long as many, and it is easy to fit into a schedule. For this method, simply have twelve hours in which you eat your day's meals and twelve hours in which you fast. This is especially great because a large portion of the fasting window can be accomplished while you sleep. For instance, if you don't eat anything after eight in the evening, you can then eat breakfast at eight in the morning.

Sixteen/Eight-Hour Fast

Also known as the Leangains diet, the sixteen/eight fast requires sixteen hours of fasting along with an eight-hour window in which you can eat your meals. If you are someone who does not get enough benefits with the twelve-hour fasting window, then you might try the sixteen/eight-hour fast.

Don't feel as if this fast has to be exactly sixteen and eight hours. Some people have difficulty fasting for longer periods and may choose a shorter fasting period. For instance, many women will choose a fourteen-hour fasting period rather than a sixteen-hour period.

People often accomplish this method of fasting simply by being careful not to eat dinner overly late in the evening and then skipping breakfast in the morning.

The sixteen/eight fast is easy to develop a habit which feels natural. People will often develop a habit where they eat on this schedule without feeling hungry, making the fast easy and simple. If you are having trouble with a longer fast, then simply try slowly increasing a shorter fast by thirty minutes until it becomes natural.

Twenty-Four-Hour Fast

One popular method of fasting, especially for men, is a once or twice weekly twenty-four-hour fast, also known as an Eat-Stop-Eat fast. Not eating for an entire day may sound difficult, but people usually do not start this type of fast until midday rather than morning, meaning that you can eat a hearty breakfast before beginning.

While you are unable to consume any calories during the fasting period, you can enjoy calorie-free beverages such as tea, coffee, and keto-approved drinks. It is important to ensure that on the non-fasting days you consume your full calorie recommendation along with plenty of nutrient-dense ingredients so that you do not become deficient in anything.

If you are afraid of a twenty-four-hour fast being more difficult, remember that fasts are easier once you are in sustained ketosis. You can also begin with a shorter fast and work your way up to a twenty-four-hour fast if you desire.

While a twenty-four-hour fast has been shown to be safe when you are consuming enough calories and nutrients on non-fasting days, it is generally better for men than women. This is because, for some women, a longer fast may interrupt their menstrual cycle.

Twice Weekly Fast

Unlike on the twenty-four-hour fast, the twice-weekly fast, while also twenty-four hours, allows you to consume some food during the fasting period. It is recommended for men to consume six-hundred calories and women to consume five-hundred calories during the fasting period. Though, just like with the twenty-four-hour fast, you can wait and begin the fasting period during midday so that you can enjoy breakfast before beginning.

It is best to separate this fast into two portions of the week, and not do them on two days back to back. For instance, rather than practicing this fast on both Monday and then Tuesday, you could follow it on Monday and Thursday.

Studies have shown that this type of fast is equally as effective for weight loss as caloric restriction, yet you are not required to restrict your caloric intake on the non-fasting days. The twice-weekly fast has also been shown to be especially powerful in improving insulin sensitivity and reducing overall insulin levels.

As you can see, there are many types of fasting you can include on the ketogenic diet. While fasting isn't a required part of the diet, there are many health benefits to including it once you have been on the ketogenic diet for at least a month and are fully adapted.

Chapter 7: Vegan, Vegetarian, or Dairy-Free Keto

Many people who choose to live a vegan or vegetarian lifestyle, or those with dairy allergies, may be concerned that the ketogenic diet might not work for them. After all, many recipes you find online will include large amounts of dairy products and meats. Some people even recommend against using low-carbohydrate soy products on the ketogenic diet.

Thankfully, it is entirely possible to be both keto and avoid these animal by-products. Whether you choose to avoid these ingredients for health, climate, or ethical reasons, you can follow a successful ketogenic diet.

Busting the Soy Myth

During the 90s, it was commonly believed that soy products, such as tofu, could cause cancer. This was believed due to scientific studies which included factors that altered the results from being completely accurate and therefore misled millions. Thankfully, as further studies have been conducted, it has been proven that not only does soy not cause cancer, but it can dramatically decrease your risk of developing this devastating disease. In fact, one study found that vegans who consume a large number of soy products are fifteen percent less likely to either develop or die of cancer.

People are also more likely to eat higher contents of fruits and vegetables when on a vegan or vegetarian ketogenic diet since they will not be using any of their daily carbohydrate count on dairy products. This is good news because the World Health Organization (W.H.O) has found that a third of cancer may be prevented by utilizing circumstances under our control. One of these circumstances is the amount of fresh produce we consume. It has been found that people who consume seven portions of fruits and vegetables daily have up to a fifteen percent decreased chance of either developing or dying of cancer.

Another study has been conducted on the soy consumption of Asian Americans and their likelihood of developing breast cancer. This study, which was conducted in Los Angeles on over a thousand Japanese, Chinese, and Filipino Americans, found that soy products do not increase the risk of cancer, but rather dramatically decrease the risk of developing cancer. In this study, the women who consumed soy at least once weekly both during adolescence and adulthood were the least likely to develop cancer. Though, the women who only consumed soy products regularly during adolescence and not adulthood were still less likely to develop breast cancer than people who never consumed soy regularly.

The Importance of Phytonutrients

As mentioned earlier, one of the benefits of a ketogenic diet without animal-derived products is that it will naturally contain more plant food. This is important, as vegetables, fruits, and other plant foods contain phytonutrients, which are a powerful bioactive non-nutrient you are unable to get from non-plant ingredients. In fact, over five-thousand types of phytonutrients have been discovered, yet scientists estimate that there are at least three-thousand more that we have yet to discover.

While we still need to learn more about these vital natural chemicals, it has been well studied and documented that they play an important role in preventing and treating a variety of the diseases that plague modern society, as well as reducing free radical production.

Epidemiological studies have shown that it is important to consume a large variety of plant foods, as the various phytonutrients that can be found in them can reduce the risk of common diseases, such as Alzheimer's, cancer, diabetes, cardiovascular diseases, neurodegenerative diseases, cataracts, and other age-related diseases. This is especially important because cancer, stroke, and heart disease are the three leading causes of death in the Western world. The fact that the Western world has also greatly reduced the servings of fruits and vegetables consumed daily may play a role in this. While it is advised to consume five to nine servings of fruits and vegetables daily, many people only consume a fraction of this.

Part of the reason that these phytonutrients can provide such a wide array of health benefits is that they are full of antioxidants. The world we live in is constantly assaulting our cells with oxidizing agents, many of which progress aging and disease. We are unable to avoid these, as they are in the air, water, food, and even produced within our own bodies during the digestion and metabolic processes. Therefore, in order to prevent a wide range of damage from oxidants, it is imperative that we also promote antioxidants.

Scientists, seeing how powerful phytonutrients are, have attempted to learn all the ways in which they can prevent and treat disease. They have even researched to attempt and find a pure version of phytonutrients which could be consumed as a pill, such as vitamins. Sadly, while this would help a great many people, at this point in time, with our current scientific understanding, it would be impossible to replicate the benefits in a purified form.

The reason for this is because when phytonutrients are consumed in a pure form, they lose their bioactive properties and no longer provide the same benefits they do when we consume them in a whole food diet. A good example of this is β-carotene. This phytonutrient is commonly found in green and yellow produce, and it contains incredible cancer-fighting and preventative properties. Yet when β-carotene has been isolated and given as a supplement, participants in studies have experienced no change. Similarly, while β-carotene has tremendous anti-cancer effects when eaten in a whole foods diet, when it was given as a supplement in a study on lung cancer mortality, the participants not only didn't experience improvement, but it may have in fact caused an adverse reaction.

While previously believed that the benefits of fruits and vegetable lied within their vitamin content, it is now known that the truly powerful benefits are not the vitamins, but rather the phytonutrients. Vitamins are great, and we require them for sound health; however, it is the phytonutrients which truly benefit us the most.

A good example is the vitamin and phytonutrient content of apples. The total antioxidant activity derived from phytonutrients in one gram of apple with the skin included is equivalent to 83.3 micromoles of vitamin C. This means that the antioxidant properties of one-hundred grams of apples are equivalent to 1500 milligrams of vitamin C. This is much higher than the antioxidant activity of vitamin C in one gram of apple, which is 0.057 milligrams. What does this indicate? The vitamin C only contributes to 0.4 percent of the antioxidant activity found in apples. Thus, most of the antioxidant properties do not come from the vitamin C, but rather from the phytonutrients.

But why are the phytonutrients powerful when eaten naturally in our diet and not when taken in a pill? The reason for this is because phytonutrients have strong synergistic effects, where the many phytonutrients which are in any given fruit or vegetable work together in order to cause the benefits they can produce. In a nutshell, they are unable to produce these benefits on their own, but only when they are eaten in conjunction.

There is an average of eight-thousand phytonutrients found in fruits and vegetables, and these all come in different sizes, solubility, and polarity. All of these differences can affect their bioavailability and which organs, tissues, cells, macromolecules, and subcellular organelles they benefit.

Rather than wasting money on a host of various nutritional supplements and vitamins, which are unlikely to make any difference in your health, it is much more effective and proactive to consume a rich diet full of a variety of fruits and vegetables. Therefore, vegan, vegetarian, or dairy-free ketogenic diets are wonderful options, as people will naturally consume more of these important fruits, vegetables, and phytonutrients.

Vegan Protein Sources:

Getting protein is simpler when you are solely dairy-free or vegetarian, as on the former you can eat meat and eggs and the latter you can still eat eggs. However, there are still some wonderful protein options for vegans and vegetarians on the ketogenic diet, though some of them may have to be eaten in moderation so that you can be mindful of your net carbohydrate intake.

Tofu

While tofu is made from beans, it is a wonderful source of protein, with many health benefits, which is also low in carbohydrates. Whether you are vegan, vegetarian, or neither, tofu can be a healthful addition to your diet. One beautiful aspect of tofu is that you can easily flavor it in many ways. You can marinate and roast firm tofu, or you could make a delicious and creamy mousse out of silken tofu.

This traditional Asian ingredient is also known as bean curd and made similarly to cheese. After soy milk is made, it is then curdled, pressed, and cooled. The liquid, otherwise known as whey, is then discarded. You can find it in many varieties for a wide range of dishes, including silken, regular, firm, extra firm, seasoned, smoked, and fermented.

Studies have been conducted on tofu, showing that it can improve cardiovascular health, lower cholesterol, reduce the risk of developing cancer, treat anemia, increase brain health, prevent osteoporosis, treat kidney disease, reduce the symptoms of menopause, prevent anemia, and increase weight loss. Tofu is also a wonderful source of protein, as it contains all of the nine essential amino acids, making an especially powerful meat substitute.

And, lest you not think that you will be depriving yourself of vitamins and minerals when eating tofu, it is actually quite high in many. Some of the vitamins and minerals it is most known for are vitamin B1, iron, calcium, selenium, phosphorous, zinc, copper, manganese, and magnesium.

Tempeh

While most soy products originated in China and its regions, tempeh is an exception that was actually invented in Indonesia. This soy product may be more difficult to find than tofu, but it is worth looking for at your nearby local Asian markets. Tempeh is made through a cultured fermentation which binds together soybeans into a heavy brick. Due to having the whole soybean, unlike tofu, tempeh is also higher in fiber, protein, vitamins, and minerals. In fact, a single serving of tempeh (30 ounces) contains only three net carbohydrates but sixteen grams of protein, and like tofu, this protein contains all of the important amino acids.

Some people may be nervous to try tempeh since it is fermented, but it has a pleasant slightly sweet and earthy flavor that tastes nutty. It also has a firm and chewy texture, which many people enjoy over the texture of tofu. While you can enjoy tempeh plain and uncooked, it is delicious when marinated, pan-fried, baked, or grilled, especially since it can absorb the flavors of whatever it is marinated in.

The nutrients in tempeh are even more amazing than tofu. It contains large amounts of calcium, riboflavin, niacin, iron, manganese, magnesium, and phosphorous. However, what is truly wonderful is that the fermentation process has its own health benefits, which many people don't consume enough of. The probiotics it gains from this can increase healthy gut bacteria, increase weight loss, prevent diarrhea, reduce bloating, improve the symptoms of irritable bowel syndrome, and increase regularity. The fermentation process will also break down the phytic acid naturally found in soybeans, which makes them more easily digested by a wide range of people.

Miso Paste

Like tempeh, miso paste is a fermented soy product with many health benefits originating both from the soybean and the fermentation project. This paste is often a condiment added to flavor many dishes, including the traditional miso soup. When using miso paste, it is best to add it after the dish has finished cooking, so that you do not cook off any of the beneficial probiotics naturally found in it. For this reason, most traditional miso soups will not add the miso until the very end.

While miso is most traditionally made with soybeans, it can be found made with other beans or peas, which are a wonderful option for people with soybean allergies.

A single serving of red soybean miso paste (one tablespoon, sixteen grams) contains four net carbohydrates and two grams of protein. It also contains high levels of vitamin K, copper, zinc, and manganese. This may not be an ideal protein to net carbohydrate ratio on the ketogenic diet, but it has many health benefits, and eaten on occasion it shouldn't be a problem.

Edamame

Edamame, otherwise known as immature soybeans, are rich in protein and important micronutrients. Unlike full grown soybeans, edamame are still in their pod which increases the fiber and therefore decreases the number of net carbohydrates they contain. Whereas full grown soybeans contain thirty-nine net carbohydrates per cup, edamame only contains seven. This serving also includes seventeen grams of protein, along with high levels of potassium and magnesium. Edamame also has decent amounts of vitamin C, vitamin B6, vitamin K, calcium, iron, and zinc.

Mung Bean Sprouts

Mung bean sprouts have been a well-loved, healthy, low-carbohydrate, and nutrient dish across East Asia for centuries. They are eaten raw in salads and sandwiches or cooked at the main component in many stir-fries. While they are widely eaten both raw and cooked, and they contain more nutrients when raw, it is important to keep in mind that sometimes they might develop bacteria that needs to be cooked off. While not generally dangerous, for this reason, it is often recommended against children, the elderly, pregnant women, or chronically ill people to eat bean sprouts unless they have first been cooked.

A single serving (one-hundred and four grams) of mung bean sprouts, which are fresh, crisp, and filling, contains three grams of protein, four net carbohydrates, and thirty-one calories. They are also high in vitamin K, vitamin C, folate, and iron.

Broccoli Sprouts

Broccoli sprouts are becoming more common and can be found in many grocery stores, but they can also easily be grown for a fraction of the price. A single four-ounce serving of broccoli sprouts contains only one net carbohydrate, two grams of protein, and thirty-five calories. They are also high in vitamin C, and vitamin A. Broccoli sprouts also contain small amounts of iron and calcium.

One amazing aspect of broccoli sprouts is that like other cruciferous vegetables they contain glucoraphanin. Although the amount they contain is ten to one-hundred times more than adult broccoli, the exact amount varies depending on how fresh it is and whether or not they are raw. This is important because glucoraphanin is a precursor to isothiocyanate, which activates enzymes that fight against the disease. Broccoli sprouts have been shown to reduce the risk of, and fight against, cancer, support detoxification, improve respiratory function, prevent cardiovascular diseases, aid in the management of multiple sclerosis, protect the brain from neurodegenerative diseases, and protect against H. pylori.

Vegan Isolated Protein Powder

There are various forms of vegan protein powder, but a recommended one is Hammer Nutrition's Vanilla Soy Protein, as it is separated from the other components of the soybean. This increases the protein level while decreasing the number of carbohydrates it contains. Despite this, it is still high in the important vitamins, minerals, and phytonutrients that we all know and love within soy. This protein powder is nutrient dense, easily absorbed by the body, and contains no sugar, artificial colors, preservatives, or GMOs.

One scoop of their vanilla soy protein powder contains one-hundred and ten calories, twenty-three grams of protein, one gram of fat, and only two net carbohydrates.

As you can see, the vegan, vegetarian, or dairy-free ketogenic diet may look a little different, but it contains many powerful benefits to your health and is maintainable.

Chapter 8: Which Foods to Enjoy and Avoid

There are many foods you can enjoy on the ketogenic diet, and it isn't difficult to remember which ones to avoid. In this chapter, we will go into detail on some of the foods that are especially helpful on the ketogenic diet and which are especially damaging to the ketosis process. While we may be unable to go into detail on every food you can eat on the ketogenic diet, don't worry. In the next chapter, you will be provided with an extensive shopping list.

Go-To Foods:

Avocados

While most people think of avocados as a vegetable, they are actually a fruit. Whether you are eating them as a whole ingredient or as avocado oil, they contain many benefits. One cup of avocado only contains two net carbohydrates, making it a wonderful option when you are trying to find something nutrient dense but are already nearing your daily allotment of net carbohydrates. They also contain twenty-one grams of fat, three grams of protein, and seven-hundred and eight grams of potassium. Be aware though; avocados are high in calories, and this serving contains two-hundred and thirty-four calories.

Avocados are high in many important vitamins and minerals, including vitamin C, vitamin B5, and B6, vitamin E, vitamin K, vitamin A, riboflavin, thiamine, niacin, iron, magnesium, manganese, copper, zinc, and phosphorous.

Olives

Olives, like avocados, are another fruit that is often not recognized as such. They also contain some of the same healthy fats as avocados, making them a wonderful source on the ketogenic diet, whether you are eating them whole or in the way of extra virgin olive oil. They can be a wonderful flavor booster to many dishes, whether you sprinkle them on top of a salad or make a tapenade.

This savory stone fruit is high in antioxidants, vitamin E, sodium, calcium, iron, and copper. Many studies have looked into the health effects of olives, and they are especially helpful when it comes to treating heart and bone health, as well as reducing your risk of developing cancer.

Mushrooms

Mushrooms have long been known to be a powerful health food. In fact, they have been used medicinally across Asia for centuries. This hearty fungus protects the immune system, prevents cellular damage, lowers cholesterol, and reduces the risk of developing cancer. They are also high in many vitamins and minerals, including B vitamins, vitamin D, potassium, selenium, and copper.

Sardines

Sardines, when packed in olive oil, are an incredibly healthy and nutritious option. Not only are they full of vital omega-3 fatty acids, but they are also a good source of protein. Some fish may be higher in mercury which can be dangerous, but due to the small size of sardines, they are one of the lowest fish in this mineral. Along with being a wonderful source of omega-3, sardines are also high in vitamin B-12, vitamin D, niacin, potassium, iron, magnesium, phosphorous, and zinc.

Salmon

Salmon, along with sardines, is one of the best sources of fatty fish. In fact, it is commonly known as one of the most nutritious foods. This tasty fish is high in omega-3 fatty acids and a wonderful source of protein. It is also high in a variety of B vitamins, potassium, selenium, and antioxidants.

Salmon has been found to help improve cardiovascular health, protects the immune system, increases cognitive function, reduces inflammation, strengthens bones, aid in weight loss, protect brain health, and helps fetal brain development during pregnancy.

Liver

Many people worry that liver may be full of harmful oxidants and other compounds because the liver is what helps remove these from the body. However, the liver is not a sieve. It doesn't catch these compounds and then hold onto them; it expels them all. Therefore, liver contains no more harmful compounds than any other meat. In fact, liver is one of the most nutritious foods.

It may seem odd adding it to your diet; after all, organ meat has largely disappeared from the Western diet as people have relied less on using every portion of meat available. However, this is a shame because by abandoning liver, we have abandoned many of the health-promoting qualities it contains. If you are nervous about eating liver, then try beginning in small quantities and combining it with other meat. You are unlikely to notice much difference.

One three and a half ounce serving of beef or chicken liver contains more than our daily requirement for B12. It is also high in vitamin A, vitamin C, folate, riboflavin, iron, copper, and choline.

Asparagus

Asparagus is a wonderful low-carbohydrate option that can be eaten in a variety of ways, whether you want it roasted or pureed into a soup. And, if you are looking for an excuse to eat bacon, look no further than pairing it with this tasty vegetable. One cup of asparagus contains only twenty-seven calories, two net carbohydrates, and three grams of protein.

Potassium is high in potassium, vitamin A, vitamin C, vitamin E, and vitamin K, as well as calcium, iron, copper, and folate. Asparagus has also been shown to improve insulin sensitivity, lower high blood sugar, protect against cancer, increase cognitive functioning, and increase urine health.

Spaghetti Squash

This squash gets its name from its uncanny resemblance to spaghetti. While it may not taste quite the same, it is delicious and will complement a wide variety of sauces in the same way that spaghetti does. A one cup serving of this squash contains thirty-one calories and five and a half net carbohydrates, making it a wonderful addition to the ketogenic diet, especially for people who don't want to give up their noodles. This squash is a wonderful source of vitamin C, B vitamins, potassium, and manganese, as well as a small amount of vitamin A. Spaghetti squash boosts skin and eye health, fights oxidative stress and free radicals, increases wound healing, decreases inflammation, improves cardiovascular health, prevents osteoporosis, and increases the health of a baby during pregnancy.

Collard Greens

You most likely heard your entire childhood about the health benefits of spinach. And, while it is true in a sense, it is also a lie. This is because spinach is high in oxalates, which is a compound that prevents your body from absorbing all of the nutrients it contains. Thankfully, other healthy greens are lower in oxalates, and the greens that are the lowest are collard greens. This delicious southern food is wonderful either raw or simmered down in bacon until tender. They are especially good to use in place of a tortilla when making wraps.

These amazing greens are high in fiber, vitamin A, vitamin E, vitamin C, vitamin K, folate, calcium, and iron, all of which is easily digestible in this form.

Grass-Fed Butter

Fats make up a large portion of the ketogenic diet, and because of this, you need to choose the best fats possible when you can. While everyone may not be able to afford grass-fed butter, such as Kerrygold, if you can, then this is the best option for butter. This is because grass-fed does not only taste much better, but it is five times higher in nutrients than typical butter.

This butter is rich in antioxidants, vitamin A, vitamin E, vitamin D, iodine, selenium, and lecithin. Grass-fed butter is also high in vitamin K2, which you are unable to get in plant-sourced fats. This type of butter has even been found to improve cardiovascular health, reduce chronic inflammation, increase weight loss, and improve eye health. Butter may be saturated fat, but grass-fed butter is full of many proven health benefits and well worth adding into your diet.

Coconut Oil

While coconut oil may have some naysayers due being a saturated fat, their criticism overlooks the hundreds upon hundreds of studies on the health-promoting benefits of coconut oil. Coconut oil has been proven to improve cholesterol, reduce the risk of cardiovascular disease, treat Alzheimer's disease, aid in weight loss, reduce seizure frequency, kill harmful microorganisms, reduce hunger cravings, increase skin and hair health, boost cognitive function, and coconut specifically targets abdominal fat, which is the most dangerous type of body fat. Coconut oil is also high in medium-chain triglycerides, which can be utilized for fuel much quicker than most oils, aiding in energy levels. The medium-chain triglycerides are also known to increase the production of ketones.

Some other great sources of coconut fat are coconut milk, coconut butter, and creamed coconut.

Sesame Seed Oil

Sesame seed oil has many amazing nutrients and healing properties, but you don't just have to use it as an oil; you can also get whole sesame seeds and tahini, though the seed oil is the most potent.

Some of the many scientifically proven benefits of sesame seed oil include lowered blood, improved rheumatoid arthritis, a lesson in anemia, strengthened bones, improved skin and oral health, and lessened stress and depression. It is also high in vitamin E and vitamin K.

Konjac Noodles

Konjac fiber, also known as glucomannan, is commonly used to make noodles and even a rice-like product. While konjac has been used for centuries in East Asia as a low-carbohydrate healthy alternative, it has only recently taken the West by storm. Thankfully, it can now be found in most supermarkets and is easy to come by. Throughout history, it has even been used in Chinese medicine to treat asthma, coughs, burns, skin disorders, breast pain, and hernias. Studies have now shown that konjac fiber can also improve the metabolism of carbohydrates, significantly lower cholesterol, and improve colon health.

The pure fiber of konjac, or glucomannan, can also be bought online for use in cooking at home. Using it this way you can make custard, sauces, and in general as a thickener. You might even try your hand at making keto-friendly Korean jelly drinks.

Almonds

You should be careful not to eat too many nuts, even though most nuts are approved. This is because the carbohydrate count in them does add up, and they are extremely high in calories. It is not uncommon for people to hit a weight loss stall, only to find that they had been eating either too many nuts or too much dairy. Although, in moderation, nuts are a wonderful and healthy addition. They are high in fiber, fat, and protein, as well as in many micronutrients, such as vitamin E, niacin, riboflavin, calcium, and antioxidants.

Chia Seeds

These seeds are highly nutritious and can be added to a number of dishes, but one of the people's favorite uses of chia seeds is to make low-carbohydrate puddings. This is an especially useful utilization of the seed, as when they absorb water and form a thick gel they can help detox your digestive tract.

This little seed is high in protein, fiber, and fat, along with vitamin B 12, thiamine, niacin, calcium, zinc, magnesium, manganese, phosphorous, and potassium.

Blackberries

While most fruit is avoided on the ketogenic diet, due to the sugar in it causing high levels of carbohydrates, berries are one of the few fruits you may enjoy in moderation. A half cup of blackberries contains six net carbohydrates, making it the perfect sweet snack when you are craving refreshing fruit. Blackberries are also high in fiber, vitamin C, vitamin K, manganese, and antioxidants. It also contains anti-inflammatory and antibacterial properties.

Keep Away Foods:

Potatoes

Yes, potatoes are a vegetable, but they are extremely high in carbohydrates. In fact, one medium white potato contains over thirty net carbohydrates, and one medium sweet potato contains about twenty-five net carbohydrates.

Grains and Beans

While a few soy products are approved on the ketogenic diet, such as tofu and edamame, otherwise beans and grains should be avoided. They all have extremely high net carbohydrate counts, despite their high fiber content.

Most Fruit

Berries are permitted in moderation and melon in moderation on occasion, but aside from that, you will want to avoid fruits, especially those that have been dried.

Cashews, Pistachios, and Chestnuts

While most nuts are low enough in carbohydrates to be allowed on the ketogenic diet, cashews, pistachios, and chestnuts are simply too high.

Milk and Low-Fat Dairy

While full-fat dairy is approved on the ketogenic diet, try to avoid milk and low-fat dairy, as both of these are higher in carbohydrates. Instead, stick with full-fat cheeses, sour cream, and whipping cream.

Natural Sweeteners

These sweeteners, even if low on the glycemic index, will still raise your blood sugar and are also high in carbohydrates.

Artificial Sweeteners

Some people may choose to partake in artificial sweeteners on the ketogenic diet, and that is their choice. However, it is not recommended due to studies showing their ill effects on health and the possibility of them affects your insulin response regardless of being zero caloric.

You may notice that stevia and erythritol are recommended on the ketogenic diet. This is because these are zero calorie and natural options that do not affect blood sugar or insulin.

Alcohol

There is alcohol that doesn't contain carbohydrates, such as vodka. However, it is still not recommended because when your body is burning off the alcohol, it will be unable to process any food or calories in your system; thereby impeding weight loss. You are also more likely to get drunk and hungover when on the ketogenic diet.

However, if you insist on having a small drink for a special occasion, then your best options would be champagne, dry wine, dry martinis, tequila, whiskey, rum, vodka, and brandy.

Chapter 9: Ketogenic Shopping List

There may be certain foods you are required to stay away from on the ketogenic diet, and this can be daunting. But that doesn't mean the ketogenic diet is difficult. There are many foods you can fully enjoy, either on the go or for a sit-down dinner. In this chapter, shopping lists are provided that you can use to plan your meals and to make it easier to know what you *can* eat, rather than what you can't eat.

Fruits and Vegetables:

1 ounce/28 grams	Arugula	0.6 net carbs	1 ounce/28 grams	Kale	2.2 net carbs
1 ounce/28 grams	Artichokes	1.4 net carbs	1 ounce/28 grams	Lemons	1.8 net carbs
1 ounce/28 grams	Asparagus	0.5 net carbs	1 ounce/28 grams	Limes	3.5 net carbs
1 ounce/28 grams	Avocados	0.5 net carbs	1 ounce/28 grams	Lingonberries	6.9 net carbs
1 ounce/28 grams	Bamboo	0.9 net	1 ounce/28 grams	Lettuce	0.3 net

grams	Shoots	carbs	grams	(Romaine)	carbs
1 ounce/28 grams	Beet Greens	0.2 net carbs	1 ounce/28 grams	Mushrooms (white)	0.6 net carbs
1 ounce/28 grams	Blackberries	1.4 net carbs	1 ounce/28 grams	Okra	1.1 net carbs
1 ounce/28 grams	Blueberries	3.4 net carbs	1 ounce/28 grams	Olives	2.2 net carbs
1 ounce/28 grams	Bok Choy	0.4 net carbs	1 ounce/28 grams	Onions (yellow)	2.1 net carbs
1 ounce/28 grams	Broccoli	1.2 net carbs	1 ounce/28 grams	Parsley	0.9 net carbs
1 ounce/28 grams	Broccoli Sprouts	0.3 net carbs	1 ounce/28 grams	Peppers (bell)	1.0 net carbs
1 ounce/28 grams	Broccolini	1.0 net carbs	1 ounce/28 grams	Pumpkin	1.7 net carbs
1 ounce/28 grams	Brussels Sprouts	1.4 net carbs	1 ounce/28 grams	Purslane	2.4 net carbs
1 ounce/28 grams	Cabbage (green)	0.9 net carbs	1 ounce/28 grams	Radicchio	1.0 net carbs
1 ounce/28 grams	Cabbage (nappa)	0.6 net carbs	1 ounce/28 grams	Radishes	0.6 net carbs
1 ounce/28 grams	Cauliflower	0.8 net carbs	1 ounce/28 grams	Raspberries	1.5 net carbs
1 ounce/28 grams	Celery	0.6 net carbs	1 ounce/28 grams	Rhubarb	3.3 net carbs
1 ounce/28 grams	Chard	0.6 net carbs	1 ounce/28 grams	Rutabaga	1.0 net carbs
1 ounce/28 grams	Collard Greens	0.7 net	1 ounce/28 grams	Spaghetti	3.9 net

grams		carbs	grams	Squash	carbs
1 ounce/28 grams	Cranberries	2.1 net carbs	1 ounce/28 grams	Spinach	0.4 net carbs
1 ounce/28 grams	Cucumbers	0.9 net carbs	1 ounce/28 grams	Strawberries	1.6 net carbs
1 ounce/28 grams	Gooseberries	1.7 net carbs	1 ounce/28 grams	Summer Squash	0.6 net carbs
1 ounce/28 grams	Daikon	0.7 net carbs	1 ounce/28 grams	Tomatoes	1.9 net carbs
1 ounce/28 grams	Dandelion Greens	1.7 net carbs	1 ounce/28 grams	Turnips	1.3 net carbs
1 ounce/28 grams	Eggplant	0.6 net carbs	1 ounce/28 grams	Turnip Greens	1.1 net carbs
1 ounce/28 grams	Endive	0.0 net carbs	1 ounce/28 grams	Watercress	0.3 net carbs
1 ounce/28 grams	Fennel	1.1 net carbs	1 ounce/28 grams	Zucchini	0.6 net carbs
1 ounce/28 grams	Green Beans	1.0 net carbs			
1 ounce/28 grams	Jicama	1.1 net carbs			

Dairy:

1 ounce/28 grams	Blue Cheese	0.7 net carbs
1 ounce/28 grams	Brie	0.1 net carbs
1 ounce/28 grams	Cheddar	0.1 net carbs

1 ounce/28 grams	Colby	0.7 net carbs
1 ounce/28 grams	Cottage Cheese (2% fat)	1.0 net carbs
1 ounce/28 grams	Cottage Cheese (creamed)	0.9 net carbs
1 ounce/28 grams	Cream Cheese	1.1 net carbs
1 ounce/28 grams	Feta	1.1 net carbs
1 ounce/28 grams	Goat Cheese (soft)	0.2 net carbs
1 ounce/28 grams	Goat Cheese (hard)	0.6 net carbs
1 ounce/28 grams	Gouda	0.6 net carbs
1 ounce/28 grams	Heavy Cream	0.8 net carbs
1 ounce/28 grams	Mozzarella (whole milk)	0.6 net carbs
1 ounce/28 grams	Parmesan	0.9 net carbs
1 ounce/28 grams	Ricotta (whole milk)	0.9 net carbs
1 ounce/28 grams	Sour Cream	0.7 net carbs
1 ounce/28 grams	Swiss	1.5 net carbs
1 ounce/28 grams	Yoghurt (plain)	1.3 net carbs

Nuts and Seeds:

1 ounce/28 grams	Almonds	2.0 net carbs
1 ounce/28 grams	Almond Butter	2.0 net carbs
1 ounce/28 grams	Almond Meal	2.0 net carbs
1 ounce/28 grams	Brazil Nuts	1.4 net carbs
1 ounce/28 grams	Chia Seeds	
1 ounce/28 grams	Golden Flaxseed (meal)	1.1 net carbs
1 ounce/28 grams	Hazelnuts	2.0 net carbs
1 ounce/28 grams	Macadamias	1.6 net carbs
1 ounce/28 grams	Pecans	1.2 net carbs
1 ounce/28 grams	Pili Nuts	1.1 net carbs
1 ounce/28 grams	Pine Nuts	2.7 net carbs
1 ounce/28 grams	Poppy Seeds	2.2 net carbs
1 ounce/28 grams	Sesame Seeds	3.3 net carbs
1 ounce/28 grams	Sesame Seed Oil	0 net carbs
1 ounce/28 grams	Sunflower Seeds	3.2 net carbs
1 ounce/28 grams	Sunflower Seed Butter (sugar-free)	1.3 net carbs
1 ounce/28 grams	Tahini	5.2 net carbs
1 ounce/28 grams	Walnuts	2.0 net carbs

Protein:

Beef	Eggs	Scallops
Chicken	Fish	Squid
Clams	Lamb	Tempeh
Crab	Mussels	Tofu
Crawfish	Octopus	Pork
Duck	Organ Meats	Sardines (packed in olive oil)
Edamame	Pheasant	

Fats:

Avocado Oil	Coconut Oil	Macadamia Oil	Olive Oil	Walnut Oil
Cocoa Butter	Lard	MCT Oil	Sesame Seed Oil	

Miscellaneous:

Greek Dressing (Primal Kitchen)	Stoka Energy Bar	Zevia soda
Ranch Dressing (Primal Kitchen)	Himalayan Salt	Zevia Energy
Balsamic Vinaigrette (Primal Kitchen)	Coconut flour	Erythritol
Caesar Dressing (Primal Kitchen)	Whey Powder (Naked Whey)	Sweet Leaf drops

Mayo (Primal Kitchen)	Konjac Noodles	Monkfruit Sweetener (Lakanto)
Coconut Aminos	Water Drops (SweetLeaf)	Electrolyte Powder (Ultima)
Exogenous Ketones (Perfect Keto)	Water Enhancer (Stur)	Dark Chocolate 70% (Lily's)
Maple Flavored Syrup (Lakanto)	Collagen Powder	Energy Pods (KetoGeek)
Energy Bars (Keto Bars)	Victoria's Marinara Sauce	Keto Kreme (Pruvit)

Chapter 10: A 21-Day Ketogenic Meal Plan

Whenever you begin a new diet, it can be difficult to know what you can eat in the beginning. After all, it is completely different from your previous way of life. In this chapter, a twenty-one-day meal plan is provided which will help make the change as smooth as possible. You won't have to wrack your brain attempting to think of anything to eat because, as you will soon learn, there are many possibilities. Many options are given, but if you want to make the diet as easy as you can, you may want to limit your meal plan to only a few select dishes which you can enjoy repeatedly.

Week One:

	Sunday	**Monday**	**Tuesday**
Breakfast	Fathead Dough Cheese Danish	Vegetable Frittata	Chocolate Almond Butter Chia Pudding
Lunch	Low-Carb Sausage Wrapped in Bacon and Roasted. Served with Mayonnaise, Primal Kitchen Salad Dressing, or	Egg Salad with Pork Rinds and a Side of Vegetables	Caesar Salad with Primal Kitchen's Dressing

	Guacamole. With a Side of Vegetables.		
Snack	Buttercream Fat Bombs	Lily's Dark Chocolate	Pork Rinds
Dinner	Thai Shrimp Curry Konjac Noodles	Jalapeno Popper Casserole	Burrito Bowls with Beef, Lettuce, Guacamole, Onions, Tomatoes, Cilantro, Cheese, and Sour Cream

	Wednesday	Thursday	Friday	Saturday
Breakfast	Fried Eggs, Bacon, and Tomatoes	Bulletproof Coffee, Breakfast Sausage, and Strawberries	Mushroom and cheese scrambled eggs	Grain-Free Pancakes
Lunch	Beef Burger with Bacon, Cheese, Mayonnaise, and Wrapped in Lettuce or Served Over a Salad	Cobb Salad with Egg, Tomato, Chicken, Bacon, Cheese, and Avocado	Tuna Salad and Avocado	Lasagna Ingredients (minus the noodles) Melted Together in a Bowl
Snack	Chocolate Chip Cookie	Matcha Fat Bombs	Chocolate Raspberry	Instant Cheesecake

			Almond Bark	Whip with Strawberries
Dinner	Hot Wings with Blue Cheese Dipping Sauce and Vegetable of Choice	Hot Dogs Without the Bun, Served with Your Favorite Toppings and a Side of Vegetables	Roasted Chicken with Asparagus and Hollandaise Sauce	Bacon and Tomato Chicken Salad in Lettuce Wraps

Week Two:

	Sunday	Monday	Tuesday
Breakfast	Cauliflower Hash Browns and Eggs	Fathead Dough Breakfast Sausage and Cheese Balls	Eggs and Cheese Rolled in Ham and Roasted
Lunch	Cream of Mushroom Soup	Chicken Beansprout Stir-Fry with Sesame Seeds	Broccoli Cheddar Cheese Soup
Snack	Mocha Fat Bombs	Cauliflower Cheddar Cheese Tots	Cauliflower Hummus with Cucumber Slices
Dinner	Sesame Chicken and Stir-Fry	Roasted Salmon with Butter and Capers	Beef Stroganoff Meatballs over Zucchini Noodles

	Wednesday	Thursday	Friday	Saturday
Breakfast	Grain-Free Chocolate Muffin in a Mug	Cottage Cheese, Bulletproof Coffee or Tea, and Berries	Bacon and Sausage Egg Bake	Grain-Free Pancake and Egg Breakfast Sandwiches
Lunch	Sardines and Tomato Salad	Cloud Bread Ham and Cheese Sandwich	Ham, Cream Cheese, Cheddar, and Pickle Wraps	Cloud Bread Grilled Cheese Sandwich
Snack	Roasted Cauliflower Bites	Cheesy Summer Squash Gratin	Almond Chocolate Fat Bombs	Deviled Eggs with Bacon
Dinner	Lemon Butter Chicken with Broccoli	Cauliflower Crust Pizza with Your Favorite Toppings	Spaghetti Squash with Bacon, Beef, Cheese, and Victoria's Marinara Sauce	Chicken Cordon Bleu with a Side Salad

Week Three:

	Sunday	Monday	Tuesday
Breakfast	Grain Free Waffles	Breakfast Sausage "Corn" Dogs wrapped in Fathead Dough	Tahini and Coconut Shake with Protein Powder and Exogenous Ketones
Lunch	Warm Cloud Bread Sandwich with Olive Tapenade, Ham, and Swiss Cheese	Vegetable Medley Soup	Creamy Chicken Soup with Cheddar Cheese
Snack	Almond Butter Chocolate Fat Bombs	Almond Crusted Mozzarella Cheese Sticks and Victoria's Marinara Sauce	Key Lime Cheesecake Fat Bombs
Dinner	Konjac Noodle Macaroni and Cheese	Roasted Brisket, Brussels Sprouts, Roasted Radishes	Eggplant Lasagna

	Wednesday	**Thursday**	**Friday**	**Saturday**
Breakfast	Grain Free Blueberry Muffins	Deviled Eggs and Avocado	Collard Green Breakfast Wrap with Egg, Cheese, and Bacon	Chocolate Waffles with Lily's Chocolate Chips and Whipped Cream
Lunch	Egg-Filled Roasted Avocados	Butternut Squash Cream Soup	Cloud Bread Grilled Cheese with Sautéed Onions and Cheese of Choice, Side of Vegetables	Kale Salad with Nuts, Blue Cheese, Blueberries, and Primal Kitchen's Dressing of Choice
Snack	Lemon Coconut Fat Bombs	Almonds and Lily's Chocolate Chips	Cheese and Nuts	Ham and Cheese Wraps
Dinner	Zucchini Noodle Shrimp Garlic Alfredo	Stuffed and Grilled Mushrooms	Roasted Fish with Cilantro, Lemon, and Coleslaw	Sesame Marinated Tofu with Bean Sprout Stir-Fry

As you can see, there is a great variety of dishes which you can enjoy on the ketogenic diet. While this menu plan is for people on the standard ketogenic diet, you can easily adapt it to be vegan, vegetarian, or dairy-free. You can also accommodate many other food allergies on this diet as well.

Chapter 11: Ketogenic Meal Prepping

One of the biggest reasons people hold off on starting a diet, even if they want to lose weight or improve their health, is because of the time it takes. If you aren't able to pick up fast food or frozen meals as easily, you can't eat whatever is just laying around. However, the ketogenic diet doesn't have to be difficult. There are many easy and quick meals you can enjoy time and time again when you are busy.

However, if you prefer a nice home-cooked meal, you can make use of meal planning and prepping in order to have a nice warm meal ready for you at the end of the day or already packaged to take to work in the afternoon.

Why Meal Plan and Prep

Planning and prepping your meals can save you a great deal of time. This is because rather than having to daily think about what you can eat, going through the pantry while both stressed and hungry and then cooking, you already have all of your food. Heat it up or put it in the crock-pot in the morning so that it will be done cooking in the evening. This also greatly limits your likelihood of falling off the wagon and eating something non-keto when hungry because you will already have all the food you need prepared.

Aside from saving you time, there are other benefits to meal planning and prepping as well. One way in which they can help is by saving your mental energy. Humans only have a certain amount of energy, both physical and mental, that we can expend in a day. Each time we have to make a choice, whether it is what to wear or what to eat, we are using up a small amount of this mental energy. This is especially true when trying to make decisions when we are tired, stressed, or hungry.

You may have heard that highly successful people often wear the same outfit every day, or otherwise limit the number of choices they have to make. That is exactly for this reason. These people limit the small ordinary decisions they can so that they can then expend their mental energy on more important matters.

If you reserve one day a week, or even every other week, to plan and prep your meals, then you can have an entire week of not having to think or make decisions about food. This will open up opportunities so that you can further your career, take care of your home, or go out and enjoy time with friends.

Believe it or not, there are still more benefits to meal planning and prepping. This method of planning ahead can save you money, which in this economy we can all benefit from. When you plan and shop once weekly, you can buy more food in bulk, shop sales, and waste less food. This is not only good for your pocketbook but the environment as well. Rather than wasting money running by a fast food restaurant or buying an expensive meal, you can plan ahead of time so that your entire week's meals fit within your set budget. To make the most of this, be sure to go through any store sale papers when doing your planning so that you can get the best deals possible.

Lastly, you can make it healthier with the correct portion size when you plan and prep ahead. No more just eating whatever "looks" like the correct amount because you will already know the exact right portion size. This will help you stay in ketosis and not eat too many or few calories. You can have a more rounded diet with a variety of vegetables and other ingredients, rather than always eating the same found. Overall, there are many benefits.

How to Plan and Prep Your Meals

To begin, you need to plan your meals. If you are looking to save as much money as possible, you will want first to look at your local sale papers and see what you can get the best deals on, and then plan a menu around those ingredients. Otherwise, you can have a list of your favorite keto meals, use the twenty-one-day meal plan in the previous chapter for inspiration, or look online for an enormous amount of delicious ketogenic recipes. Thankfully, more people have discovered the benefits of the ketogenic diet, meaning there are plenty of recipes and resources to make the process easier.

After you find some favorite ketogenic recipes, be sure that you save them. You could create a bookmarks folder, a Pinterest board, or use an online recipe book. Whatever you choose, you want to ensure that you never lose track of your favorite recipes.

When planning your meals, it can help to keep things simple. You don't want to over plan and give yourself too many meals to prep. Therefore, start with a few meals for each meal type that are easy to prepare. You want to choose meals that you wouldn't mind eating two or three times a week. Then, if you can handle prepping that amount, you can increase the variety of meals in a week.

Remember to track your macros. When you create a plan for a day, you don't want to do a bunch of high-carbohydrate dishes on the same day; otherwise, you will go over your carbohydrate limit. Use online nutrition calculators to ensure that your full day's plan is within your macro ratio. Keep an eye on the micro ratio as well, ensuring that you get enough vitamins and minerals.

One of the benefits of this is that you will then not have to worry about weighing and measuring all of your food on a day-to-day basis. You will only have to do this one day a week, or every other week, during the prep stage, and then you are set to go.

After you have your plan made, you need to find a day in which you can shop every week. If you can shop the same day, this is the best because you need to ensure that you always have meals planned and prepped, and if you go shopping later than usual, then you won't have food ready. Though, you could always account for this by having some homemade meals in the freezer for emergencies and busy times. If shopping is difficult due to time constraints, many stores are now offering to deliver your groceries directly to your car, saving you potentially hours in time.

After shopping, you should immediately put away the groceries and prepare the fresh fruits and vegetables. This will not only make the cooking process easier, but it will also keep your produce fresh for longer. Many containers promote the longevity of freshness in fruits and vegetables. You don't want to plan to use strawberries and lettuce later in the week, only for them to rot in the meantime.

During this process, you can also marinate or brine any meats or tofu that might need it. This way it will be ready to cook when you are preparing the meals.

It will greatly reduce your cooking time if you practice cooking multiple items simultaneously. Multitasking in the kitchen is extremely important to work efficiently. For instance, if you have a chicken roasting in the oven, you might also be able to roast vegetables or tofu at the same temperature.

Or, if you are cooking a sauce on the stove, why not cook other things on the stove at the same time? In this way, you can spend less time watching the food while it cooks, as you won't have to do it time and time again. This also helps because if some dishes require the same ingredients, you won't have to get them out of the fridge and put them away again multiple times – you can use it all at once.

Once your food precooked dishes are prepped, you can portion them out into proportioned containers. This is especially helpful if you are the only person eating these dishes or if you want to eat them on the go. If you are only preparing the dishes on one day and plan to cook them the next day, then you can easily store them in a large container until you plan to utilize them. This can be especially helpful for freezer meals.

Helpful Equipment:

There is a lot of equipment that can help a kitchen run more efficiently, helping you complete your task in a time-saving manner. While it is impossible to list every tool, you might need, for instance, a spatula or wooden spoon. The following will introduce you to some specific items that can make the food prep lifestyle more manageable.

Planner

You will want a good quality planner that is easy for you to plan your meals in, shopping lists, macro ratios, and a to-do list to prepare the meals. There is an abundance of planners on the market, and you can get whatever suits your style the most. However, something plain and even blank might be the most productive for this. You can get inexpensive notebooks for this purpose, but if you want to go all out, you can get a bullet journal. These are really popular in the planner community for good reason.

They are completely customizable, and they are a handy size. They are large enough to fit your needs but small enough to easily fit into a bag and be taken on the go.

Glass Storage Containers

These storage containers may be more expensive than their plastic counterparts, but they are healthier, better for the environment, hold up to heavy food, and don't stain. These glass containers have become much more popular for good reason. You can even cook portioned sized food in them, meaning fewer dishes to clean!

Plastic Storage Containers

While the glass containers are superior, it's a good idea to keep some large plastic containers on hand as well. This can come in handy when you want to freeze liquids such as homemade stock or broth. If you put stock in a glass container and then freeze it, the frozen liquid will slightly expand, causing the glass to shatter potentially. These also tend to stack really well and can hold frozen meals.

For this reason, it's preferable to use glass containers in the fridge and plastic containers in the freezer.

Glass Jars

These glass jars come in a large variety of sizes and can even be used for canning – if you are into that. They are especially convenient for storing stock, cold brew coffee, and sauces in the refrigerator. It is best to buy these in their various sizes, as the tiny ones can come in handy when you only have a small amount of sauce to store, and the large ones can help when you have stock or cold brew coffee to store.

Food Processor

Whether you need food thickly sliced, finely diced, shredded, or thickly purred, then a food processor can save you a great deal of time. No more struggling over shredding a brick of cheese with a hand-held grater. No more risking the safety of your fingers with a knife. Food processors can save you time, energy, and potentially prevent blood loss. They come in a variety of sizes. You can get large ones appropriate for ricing an entire head of cauliflower, or small ones which work well on a single small onion.

Blender

Blenders are wonderful when you want a smoothie, shake, smooth sauce, or a creamed soup. While you may want to splurge, and get the high-end Vitamix, which is an amazing all-purpose tool, there are many inexpensive decent brands. You don't have to spend a fortune to get a high-quality blender. The KitchenAid, Oster, and

Ninja blenders are all high quality and have price points which can accommodate most budgets.

Immersion Blender

Sometimes you need soup or sauce blended, but don't want to go through the trouble of getting the entire blender dirty or transferring a hot liquid into the blender. You also have to be extremely careful when blending hot liquids, as they could spray out the top of the blender, or even worse, cause the blender to shatter. Thankfully, with an immersion blender, you don't have these problems. Using one is as simple as plugging it into an outlet and stirring it around your pot, just as you would with a spoon.

Vegetable Spiralizer

These spiralizers are a wonderful tool for anyone who is on a healthy whole-food diet, and that includes people following the ketogenic lifestyle. You can simply attach a vegetable onto the spiralizer, and within seconds, you will have homemade vegetable noodles. You can also buy vegetables pre-spiralized at the store when you are trying to save energy but know that they mark the price up.

The most popular and versatile vegetable to turn into noodles is zucchini. These become a delicious noodle that you can make pasta and soups with – you can even make a satisfying stove-top macaroni and cheese with bacon!

Pressure Cooker

While pressure cookers used to be difficult to use, there are now electric pressure cookers that have taken the world by storm, and for good reason. These pressure cookers are extremely easy to use, safe, and speed up cooking by two thirds to three-quarters of the time it would otherwise take. They can also act as a crock-pot and keep your food warm after it is finished cooking. The most popular and beloved brand is Instant Pot, but many others have similar features, such as one by Hamilton, and another by Gourmia.

Crock-Pot

These are a wonderful tool, especially for anyone with a busy lifestyle who is always on the go, which let's not kid ourselves, is almost everyone. With a crock-pot, you can easily place a frozen or refrigerated meal that you previously prepped inside of the liner and allow it to cook all day on low or turn it on high a few hours before dinner for a delicious and fresh meal. This is especially helpful for people who have a job, but still want to come home to a warm freshly cooked dinner.

Large Skillet

Whether you choose to use non-stick, stainless steel, or cast iron, it doesn't matter. However, you do need a good quality large skillet that can handle cooking a large amount of food at once. If you are used to only cooking for yourself, then you might not have a large skillet, but it is important when meal prepping that you have enough space in the pan to cook multiple meals simultaneously.

Baking Sheet

These come in a variety of sizes, and it doesn't really matter which one you get as long as it has a flat base and is large. Again, you want something large enough to cook a lot of food on simultaneously. On the other hand, it could also be useful to have a few mini baking sheets on hand so that if you want to cook a single burger patty or anything else in a small serving, you won't get a large pan dirty.

Glass 9x13-inch Pan

These pans are wonderful for roasting chicken, making a large keto cake, and roasting vegetables. Really, the possibilities in how you can use one of these pans are endless. You can even find some with lids which makes it easy to roast a dish in this and then store it in the fridge in the same pan for later in the week.

Non-Stick Mats and Parchment Paper

These two supplies are endlessly helpful. The last thing you want after cooking a dish is to find it stuck to the pan. These not only prevent food from sticking, but they also make the dishes easier to clean. The non-stick mats are typically made of silicone and can be used many times, but the parchment paper can only be used once. Though, it is helpful to have both on hand because while parchment paper isn't as economical or environmental, it can be cut to the exact size of the pan.

Metal Cooling Rack

These cooling racks are often used for baked goods, such as cookies. You can remove cookies from the pan as soon as they are done cooking and allow them to cool on the rack so that the bottoms of the cookies don't burn. However, these racks also have many other uses. For instance, you can place one (with the legs folded) onto a baking sheet and then place bacon on the rack. This helps the bacon cook evenly and quickly in the oven.

Digital Kitchen Scale

A digital kitchen scale is a must-have on the ketogenic diet. Simply measuring your food is often unreliable, especially when it comes to measuring fruits and vegetables. Since they do not sit in a measuring cup evenly, as almond flour does, you don't have a correct idea of exactly how much you are eating. But with a digital scale, you can know just how many grams, ounces, or pounds a given ingredient is. This will give you much more control over your macro ratio, potentially aiding in your weight loss.

Large Cutting Board

When you are meal prepping, it will really pay off to have a large cutting board. You don't want to use a plate, as when cutting a large item, it just is too awkward and small. The counter, on the other hand, is covered in germs, and even if you clean it, the last thing you want to place on your counter is chicken. This will only give you, and everyone else, salmonella poising. A simple plastic cutting board works best, as salmonella and other bacteria will absorb into both wooden and bamboo cutting boards.

Large Chef Knife

You want a high-quality, extremely sharp and well-cared-for knife. If the blade of a knife becomes dull, then it can slip and is more likely to cause injury. Even if you can only afford one high-quality knife, try to get one large chef knife. These are especially helpful for cutting into squash, such as spaghetti or acorn squash, which is notoriously hard to cut open.

Hand Peeler

You don't want to rely on a knife to peel all of your produce, as you are more likely to injure yourself. Rather, try to find an ergonomic hand-held peeler which is sharp enough. This will also save you time because most people can peel with a peeler much quicker than with a knife.

Bento Boxes

These boxes, named 'bento' in Japanese, have become increasingly popular in Western countries. They are incredibly useful as they tend to have multiple compartments that you can include different foods in, are a perfect size, and you can easily wash them out and reuse them. There are an amazing amount of bento boxes, especially if you look online, so it is not difficult to find one that best suits your needs. These will greatly help anyone who ever needs to eat on the go, whether you need lunch at work or a snack between running errands.

Reusable Plastic Utensils

While you could just use disposable plastic utensils, these are not good for the environment. Having some reusable and lightweight utensils, that you can keep with your bento, will make it much easier to eat on the go, no matter if you are at a park, in your car, or at the office.

Insulated Bag

You can find insulated bags and small ice chests at most stores. If you place a few reusable ice packs in these, they will keep your food cold for hours. This is the perfect way to take food on the go with you without risking bacteria. This will greatly help anyone who has to be away from home for any length of time and doesn't want to have to risk going out for food. It is as easy as making a keto bento and storing it until you get hungry.

While all of these tools are helpful, you don't have to have all of them to practice meal planning and prepping. Sure, a pressure cooker saves time in cooking, but if you don't have the funds, it won't ruin your experience. The tools listed here are meant to help and guide you, not limit you.

Chapter 12: Keto FAQ

While the ketogenic diet is relatively simple and easy, it is perfectly normal to have questions when you are beginning a new diet and lifestyle. In this chapter, most common questions will be answered.

Do I Have to Track My Macros?

Yes. When you have been on the ketogenic diet for a long time, you may be able to go without tracking your macros every day, but it is especially important to track everything at the beginning. If you don't, you will likely get more net carbohydrates than you realize, and have a difficult time entering and maintaining ketosis. It is also important to track if you are trying to lose weight because fats are high in calories and you can accidentally get more than you realize. Lastly, it is essential that your body has enough protein to maintain its lean muscle mass, and if you aren't tracking your macros, you won't know if you have eaten enough.

Why Am I Not Losing Weight?

The most common reason for a weight plateau is because people stopped tracking their macros. Two of the other more common reasons are either too many dairy products or too many nuts. Try to enjoy these two items in moderation and balanced out with plenty of high fiber and low starch vegetables.

Is the Ketogenic Diet a Fad?

No, the ketogenic diet is not a fad. There is nearly a century's worth of scientific studies on the ketogenic diet due to its health promoting and brain-protecting properties. While it was originally designed for epilepsy, doctors have discovered many more uses for it, one of which is weight loss.

Is the Ketogenic Diet Safe?

Yes, in general, the ketogenic diet is extremely safe, and this has been proven throughout many scientific studies. This has been shown to be true both when the ketogenic diet is used for a short time and when it is used for a long-term solution.

While some people may experience 'keto flu' symptoms, these are not dangerous, as long as the person stays hydrated and consumes electrolytes. Although, it is best for people with kidney disease to avoid this, as well as people who are pregnant or breastfeeding. If you have a disease or chronic illness, please discuss any dietary changes with your doctor.

Is the Low-Carb Diet the Same as the Ketogenic Diet?

While the ketogenic diet is a low carbohydrate diet, this is not true the other way around. This is because low-carbohydrate diets do not have the same proportions of macros as the ketogenic diet. For instance, the low carbohydrate diet can allow up to fifty to sixty net carbohydrates a day, whereas this is double what is allowed to remain in ketosis.

My Doctor Wants me to Gain Weight, is the Ketogenic Diet for Me?

Yes! The ketogenic diet works for people no matter their weight goals. In order to lose weight on the ketogenic diet, you simply want to eat a small calorie deficit. The same is true if you need to gain weight. You simply add in the number of calories that is recommended for your weight and body type in order to gain weight, or if your doctor recommended a certain number of calories, you could use that as a guideline.

How Long Does It Take to Get into Ketosis?

The length of time it takes to enter ketosis differs for everyone. Some people may enter light ketosis within one or two days, whereas people with insulin resistance may take up to a week. After a few days in light ketosis, you should enter sustained ketosis, in which your body is producing the most effective forms of ketones. This often takes one to two weeks. Although, it can take up to a month to fully adjust to the ketogenic diet and receive increased energy levels.

How Many Carbohydrates Can I Eat?

Twenty-five to thirty is the usual recommendation, though people on the Targeted Ketogenic Diet may include an added thirty net carbohydrates before a workout. Some people will also have an even lower carbohydrate count, as low as ten net carbohydrates, in order to enter ketosis quicker.

How Long Can I Stay on the Ketogenic Diet?

Studies have shown that the ketogenic diet is safe for the long term, and there are usually no side effects after the person is fully adapted to being in ketosis. Though, while it is safe for the long term, some people choose to combine the ketogenic and Paleo diets after they reach their goal weight. This way they can remain on a healthy diet that is a little more forgiving than either the ketogenic or Paleo diets alone.

How Do I Combat Fatigue During the Keto Flu?

Thankfully, the keto flu does not last long, and some people may not even experience one. However, if you are one of the unlucky people to feel fatigue and other symptoms, as a result of making such a large change in your diet, there are ways you can decrease the symptoms.

You will want to make sure you eat more regularly, avoid fasting, and don't have too large of a calorie deficit. Remember: if you want to lose weight, you can always decrease your calorie count after week one or two.

Secondly, try to add coconut oil and MCT oil into your diet. MCT oil is pure medium-chain triglycerides, whereas coconut oil is about fifty percent medium-chain triglycerides. These shorter chain fatty acids can be absorbed and utilized by the liver for energy much quicker than other types of fat. If you are feeling a lull, then eating a fat bomb that contains either coconut oil or MCT oil can boost your energy quickly.

Be sure that you are eating your full protein macro ratio, and when you do, spread it out over the course of a day. Protein greatly increases energy levels, and if you are not eating enough, your body will begin to convert your muscle mass into energy instead.

What Should My Ketone Levels Be?

People with neurological and neurodegenerative diseases, such as Alzheimer's or epilepsy, may want higher levels of ketones. This is because ketones protect the brain from the disease. However, many people on the ketogenic diet who are healthy may obsess over their ketone levels because it's been perpetrated that your ketone level should be as high as possible. This is not true. Unless you have a neurological disease, there is no benefit of having an especially high ketone level.

As long as your ketone level is within the ketosis state (0.5 mmol/L or above), then you will be receiving the benefits of ketones. More ketones won't help you lose weight. It is also important to remember that overtime breath and urine ketone testers will become less accurate, as your body becomes more efficient in creating ketones. The most accurate way in which to test your ketone levels is with a blood ketone test.

Why Do I Have Headaches?

The most common cause for headaches is dehydration. Due to carbohydrates binding to water molecules, when you go on a low-carbohydrate diet, your body will expel these molecules, leaving you dehydrated and deficient in important electrolytes. This can also cause fatigue.

Thankfully, there is a simple solution to this. Try to drink at least half of your body weight in ounces of water every day. Even more water than this, about a gallon, is better. But make sure that you never drink more than a liter of fluids within an hour, or else your liver will be unable to handle the workload.

While you are rehydrating, it is important to also refuel on electrolytes. If you only rehydrate, then your electrolytes will only become even further out of balance. There are several ketogenic-approved electrolyte drink mixes on the market, such as Ultima Replenisher. However, you can also get pills and capsules that contain electrolytes. They should contain sodium, magnesium, potassium, and calcium.

You should increase your water and electrolyte intake further if you are doing an activity that causes you to sweat a lot, as when you sweat, you are losing both fluids and electrolytes.

Conclusion

Thank you for reading The Keto Diet: The Ultimate Ketogenic Diet Guide for Weight Loss and Mental Clarity, Including How to Get into Ketosis, a 21-Day Meal Plan, Keto Fasting Tips for Beginners and Meal Prep Ideas.

It should have given you the mental clarity you need to attain your goals. Whether your goal is to lose weight, improve your health, or even gain weight, the ketogenic diet is a simple and viable solution. There may be many fad diets out there, making it hard to know what diet you can trust, but the ketogenic diet has a century of proven results and science behind it.

Unlike diets that claim to help you lose twenty-five pounds in two weeks, only to end up gaining the weight right back, the ketogenic diet can help you lose weight healthily. You won't wreck your metabolism with this diet. Instead, you can lose weight at a maintainable pace and then keep it off.

If you choose to pair the ketogenic diet with intermittent fasting, you will find that not only is fasting easier when on the ketogenic diet, since your body has ketones to sustain itself, but you will also receive a number of health benefits.

While vegans, vegetarians, and those with dairy allergies may be concerned about the ketogenic diet, it is entirely possible to fit your needs and beliefs into this lifestyle. You may see people posting an abundance of pictures with cheese, bacon, and butter, but the ketogenic diet does not require these things. As long as you can eat fat, you can follow the ketogenic diet. This includes healthy fats, such as avocado, olive, coconut, sesame, and more.

Check out another book by Elizabeth Moore

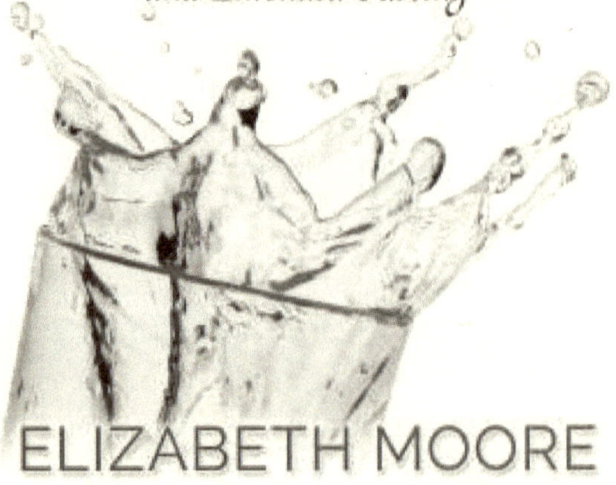